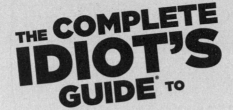

THE COMPLETE IDIOT'S GUIDE® TO

Thyroid Disease

by Dr. Alan Christianson and Hy Bender

ALPHA

A member of Penguin Group (USA) Inc.

ALPHA BOOKS

Published by the Penguin Group

Penguin Group (USA) Inc., 375 Hudson Street, New York, New York 10014, USA

Penguin Group (Canada), 90 Eglinton Avenue East, Suite 700, Toronto, Ontario M4P 2Y3, Canada (a division of Pearson Penguin Canada Inc.)

Penguin Books Ltd., 80 Strand, London WC2R 0RL, England

Penguin Ireland, 25 St. Stephen's Green, Dublin 2, Ireland (a division of Penguin Books Ltd.)

Penguin Group (Australia), 250 Camberwell Road, Camberwell, Victoria 3124, Australia (a division of Pearson Australia Group Pty. Ltd.)

Penguin Books India Pvt. Ltd., 11 Community Centre, Panchsheel Park, New Delhi—110 017, India

Penguin Group (NZ), 67 Apollo Drive, Rosedale, North Shore, Auckland 1311, New Zealand (a division of Pearson New Zealand Ltd.)

Penguin Books (South Africa) (Pty.) Ltd., 24 Sturdee Avenue, Rosebank, Johannesburg 2196, South Africa

Penguin Books Ltd., Registered Offices: 80 Strand, London WC2R 0RL, England

Copyright © 2011 by Dr. Alan Christianson

International Standard Book Number: 978-1-61564-054-6
Library of Congress Catalog Card Number: 2010910367

13 12 11   8 7 6 5 4 3 2 1

Interpretation of the printing code: The rightmost number of the first series of numbers is the year of the book's printing; the rightmost number of the second series of numbers is the number of the book's printing. For example, a printing code of 11-1 shows that the first printing occurred in 2011.

Printed in the United States of America

Most Alpha books are available at special quantity discounts for bulk purchases for sales promotions, premiums, fund-raising, or educational use. Special books, or book excerpts, can also be created to fit specific needs.

For details, write: Special Markets, Alpha Books, 375 Hudson Street, New York, NY 10014.

Publisher: *Marie Butler-Knight*

Associate Publisher: *Mike Sanders*

Senior Managing Editor: *Billy Fields*

Executive Editor: *Randy Ladenheim-Gil*

Development Editor: *Megan Douglass*

Senior Production Editor: *Janette Lynn*

Copy Editor: *Sonja Nikkila*

Cover Designer: *William Thomas*

Book Designer: *William Thomas, Rebecca Batchelor*

Indexer: *Johnna Vanhoose Dinse*

Layout: *Ayanna Lacey*

Proofreader: *John Etchison*

Alan dedicates this book to Kirin, Celestina, and Ryan.

Hy dedicates this book to the wonderful members of his movie workshop NYScreenwriters.org.

Contents

Appendixes

Introduction

One out of 10 Americans is estimated to have thyroid disease. That's over 30 million people—more than have diabetes. In contrast to other widespread illnesses, though, thyroid disease is a quiet epidemic. Many who suffer from it don't even realize they have it. That's because the thyroid regulates the energy level of your every cell; so when it malfunctions, you can develop problems involving any part of your body, including your brain, heart, bones, skin, nails, and hair.

For example, if you have hypothyroidism—caused by your thyroid becoming underactive—you may find yourself gaining weight, feeling fatigued, growing confused, becoming depressed, developing rough skin, losing hair, feeling cold, getting acne, or experiencing any of dozens of other issues.

Alternatively, if you have hyperthyroidism—caused by your thyroid becoming overactive—you may start losing weight, feeling manic, growing anxious, getting panic attacks, having trouble sleeping, developing hand tremors, sweating excessively, developing eye problems, growing goiters in your neck, or experiencing your heart pound in your chest.

Thyroid disease symptoms can creep up on you so subtly and gradually that it takes months before you even recognize that you're ill. In fact, it often isn't until patients are treated and made healthy again that they realize all the ways their bodies had gone wrong. It's for this reason that some have called thyroid disease insidious.

Thyroid disease can be hard to diagnose, even by experienced doctors. Adding to the confusion are heated debates about how to interpret lab results, which medications are most appropriate, and so on.

If you're experiencing thyroid disease symptoms and aren't sure what's causing them, this book is for you. It will guide you in identifying your symptoms, finding the right doctor, and getting the best testing and diagnosis possible.

Alternatively, if you already know that you have thyroid disease but are unsatisfied with your treatment, this book is very much for you as well. It will tell you how to analyze your lab results, choose the best medication, find the perfect dosage, and more.

Then again, if you have a friend or loved one with thyroid disease, this book will help you understand the pain it can cause, and provide you with the information to help.

Whatever the reason you need thyroid information, this book will empower you to cut through the confusion, make informed choices, and embark on the path to full health.

How to Use This Book

The first four chapters of this book apply to everyone, and we recommend that you read them first. After that, you can skip around and focus on only the chapters that most interest you. There are plentiful cross-references to chapters throughout the book, so if you encounter a term or concept that's unfamiliar you'll know which chapter to read to learn more about it.

This book's topics are organized into six parts:

Part 1, Getting to Know Your Thyroid, explains what your thyroid does and why it's so important to your health. It also describes symptoms that may indicate you have thyroid disease, controversies about thyroid diagnosis and treatment, and how to find a great doctor.

Part 2, Hypothyroidism, details what to do if you're suffering from a shortage of thyroid hormones. You'll learn what causes hypothyroidism and what diseases resemble it. You'll also learn how to recognize its symptoms, get the right tests for it, analyze your lab results, choose the right medication, and arrive at the perfect dosage to restore you to full health.

Part 3, Hyperthyroidism, describes what to do if you're suffering from an excess of thyroid hormones. You'll discover how to recognize hyperthyroidism symptoms, get the right tests for it, analyze your lab results, and choose among the different treatments for it.

Part 4, Other Thyroid-Related Diseases, provides a step-by-step guide to dealing with thyroid cancer; managing thyroid-related problems such as adrenal gland disease and parathyroid disease; and recognizing ailments such as depression, anxiety, infertility, and severe PMS that can stem from a malfunctioning thyroid.

Part 5, Diet and Lifestyle, covers food and lifestyle choices you can make to strengthen your thyroid, lose weight, shed fat, avoid toxins, and improve your overall health.

Extra Tidbits

Scattered throughout this book are sidebars designed to provide additional insights and information. They're organized into the following five categories:

THYROIDIAN TIP

Advice intended to be especially useful to you.

CRASH GLANDING

A warning or cautionary note.

THYROID FACTOID

Information you may find interesting or fun.

THROAT QUOTE

A quotation related to the subject that provides another perspective, or a laugh.

DEFINITION

Highlights a key term. (You can also find numerous definitions in Appendix A.)

Please note that this book was written by two people, Dr. Alan Christianson and Hy Bender, so the word "we" is used when advice is coming from both of us. When describing Alan's personal experiences as a doctor, though, "I" is used instead.

Please also note that this book contains a number of stories about Alan's patients to bring the medical information to life. While the stories are all true, the names and select details have been changed to protect patient privacy.

Acknowledgments

Dr. Alan Christianson: I would like to thank my closest friends who encouraged me to complete this book, with a special thanks to Ron Baron. Thanks also to my patients who encouraged me, as well as educating me every day by sharing their experiences and things they have learned. I greatly appreciate my parents who instilled a love of reading and of medicine in me at an early age, and continue to guide me. I'd also like to thank another parent, David Frawley, who as an author has given me valuable direction and insight.

Thanks to my precious children, Celestina and Ryan. Thank you both so much for being patient when I took time for this book. I love you both, and I'm so excited to see you grow into such amazing people. Biggest thanks of all go out to my lovely wife Kirin who encouraged me to pursue my dreams, and was also gracious in sharing my time with the book. My biggest wish is that all of her dreams will come true. I love you, honey!

Hy gives his heartfelt thanks to the friends who generously provided support during his struggles with thyroid cancer and hypothyroidism, including Adira Amram, Brendan Beseth, Micah Bucey, Ashley Wren Collins, Allan Fair, Kevin Hall, John Harlacher, Ada Lee Halofsky, Elena K. Holy, Ken Houghton, Sean Jaffe, Eileen Kelly, David Kempski, Margie Kment, Faye Lane, Andrew Lobel, Julie Lynch, Megan Raye Manzi, Ken Salikof, Tracey Siesser, Ken Simon, Lisa Snellings, Mark von Sternberg, Daryn Strauss, Diane Stredicke, Mariah Wilson, and Meredith Zinner; and to his surgeons, Dr. Mark Smith and Dr. William Portnoy, and his endocrinologist Dr. Maria Tulpan.

Hy also thanks the many performers in the NYC comedy community whose bravery and brilliance helped him heal more than they can know. They include (but are by no means limited to) Leo Allen, Kevin Allison, Mary Theresa Archbold, Elna Baker, Andy Christie, Johnny Conroy, Death by Roo Roo, Jessica Delfino, Amanda Duarte, Ophira Eisenberg, Fearsome, Jon Friedman, Janeane Garofalo, Christina Gausas, Chris Gethard, Leslie Goshko, Amy Heidt, Ed Herbstman, Seth Herzog, Dave Hill, Pete Holmes, Anthony Jeselnik, Anthony King, Nick Kroll, Marc Maron, Kate McKinnon, John Oliver, Lennon Parham, Sean Patton, Justin Purnell, Charlie Sanders, Kristen Schaal, Livia Scott, Paul Scheer, Blaine Swen, and Brooke Van Poppelen—all of whom proved the best medicines are laughter and love.

Trademarks

All terms mentioned in this book that are known to be or are suspected of being trademarks or service marks have been appropriately capitalized. Alpha Books and Penguin Group (USA) Inc. cannot attest to the accuracy of this information. Use of a term in this book should not be regarded as affecting the validity of any trademark or service mark.

Getting to Know Your Thyroid

1

In this part, we explain what your thyroid does, why it's vitally important to your health, and the ways it can go wrong. We also provide a checklist of thyroid disease symptoms so you can decide whether you have reason to suspect a thyroid problem.

Chapter 3 sheds light on various debates about thyroid diagnosis and treatment. And Chapter 4 guides you in finding a great doctor, and in knowing what to expect from your office visits.

Spotlighting Your Thyroid

In This Chapter

- How your thyroid regulates your cells
- Your metabolism and RMR
- Understanding thyroid hormones
- Common thyroid diseases

Thyroid disease has become a quiet epidemic. The American Association of Clinical Endocrinologists (AACE) estimates 1 in 10 Americans have thyroid disease. That's over 30 million people—more than the number of Americans with diabetes. Women are over five times as likely to have thyroid disease as men. And the chances of having a thyroid disorder increase with time—17 percent if you're a woman and 9 percent if you're a man by the time you reach age 60.

The AACE also estimates that half of those with thyroid disease don't know it. That's because thyroid issues can be difficult to recognize, even by doctors. Many people suffer from thyroid problems for years before being accurately diagnosed. Further, even if you're receiving treatment for thyroid disease, there's a strong chance you're being underserved, because many doctors rely too much on lab results and not enough on patient symptoms.

As alarming as the number of cases already is, the thyroid disease rate is expected to increase due to the thyroid's special issues with environmental toxins. The good news is that almost all thyroid disease is thoroughly treatable. The challenge is to be fully informed so you're empowered to recognize a problem and seek the right kind of help.

This chapter will take the mystery out of your thyroid. We'll explain what your thyroid is, what it does, and how it can go wrong. Whether you only suspect you have thyroid disease or are certain of it, you'll end up with the knowledge you need to start making informed choices and take appropriate next steps.

The Butterfly in Your Neck

Your *thyroid* is a butterfly-shaped gland that resides in your neck. It's wrapped around your windpipe, just above your collarbone and below your Adam's apple. Its name stems from the Greek word for "shield" (another metaphor for its shape).

 DEFINITION

The **thyroid** is a gland in your neck that behaves like your body's thermostat, raising or lowering the amount of activity taking place based on your current needs. Your thyroid affects every part of your body by secreting hormones into your bloodstream. These hormones then charge up your cell's internal power batteries, which are called mitochondria.

Your thyroid consists of left and right "wings," called *lobes*, connected by a middle section called the *isthmus*. Your thyroid's two lobes do the same job, each performing half of the necessary labor. They also effectively back each other up; if anything ever goes wrong with one lobe, the other can take over the entire workload.

The thyroid's shape varies by gender. If you're a man, it's narrower and thicker; if you're a woman, longer and flatter. That's why the Adam's apple tends to be visible in men only. Women have an Adam's apple, too—it's merely the cartilage between your thyroid and larynx—but the shape of the thyroid typically hides it from sight. (In fact, some ancient Greeks believed the purpose of the thyroid was to provide women with a pleasing neckline.)

Your thyroid isn't very large; it's roughly the width and thickness of four credit cards stacked on top of each other, and weighs 10-30 grams (0.35-1.06 ounces). Despite its relatively small size, though, your thyroid plays a critical role in your life.

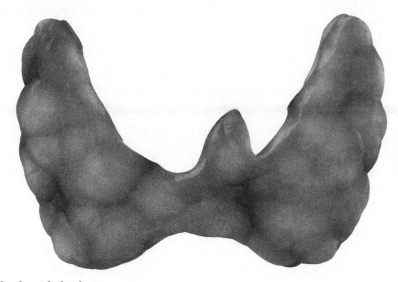

The thyroid gland.
(Licensed from Shutterstock Images)

Your Energy Control Center

The thyroid has just one job, but it's of immense importance: it makes hormones that regulate the energy level, growth, and reproduction of every cell of your body. That means your brain, heart, lungs, liver, skin, tissues, and all other body parts depend on your thyroid to stay "powered up" and active, and to remain healthy by generating new cells to replace old ones.

THYROID FACTOID

Your thyroid is one of the glands in your body's *endocrine system.* That means it secretes a chemical, or *hormone,* directly into your bloodstream that regulates targeted areas of your body. The main difference between your thyroid and most other glands is that its target is *every cell* in your body.

More specifically, each of your cells contains "power plants" called *mitochondria*. Simple cells contain just one, while more complex cells can contain several thousand mitochondria. Mitochondria take glucose (a fundamental sugar your body creates from the food you eat) and convert it into energy called *adenosine triphosphate*, or *ATP*. The cell then uses the ATP to fuel its activities (such as repairing your body, moving your body, firing thoughts in your brain, or reproducing).

How much or how little glucose the mitochondria convert into ATP is determined by the thyroid hormones circulating in your bloodstream. These hormones have a similar effect to your foot on a car's gas pedal, sending a message to either speed up or slow down. The mitochondria then function as little engines that convert your gasoline (glucose) into power (ATP) for driving your car (body).

The decisions about when to raise or lower cellular activity come from a portion of your brain called the *hypothalamus*. When your hypothalamus senses more energy is needed, it sends a chemical signal to an organ just above your sinuses that's about the size of a pea. This organ is called the *pituitary gland*.

Your pituitary gland then responds by producing *thyroid stimulating hormone*, or *TSH*. As its name indicates, TSH stimulates your thyroid, effectively telling it "We need more power. Get to work and make more hormones." Your thyroid then complies, making its hormones available to the mitochondria in each of your cells.

DEFINITION

Thyroid stimulating hormone (TSH) is the chemical regulator of your thyroid. When your body needs more energy, your pituitary gland secretes TSH, which spurs your thyroid to produce hormones. TSH is also an important diagnostic tool, because measuring its levels in your blood helps a doctor determine whether your thyroid is making too little of its hormones (TSH will be high) or too much (TSH will be low).

You can think about this energy management system as a company. The hypothalamus is the president, making "big picture" decisions about when to increase or decrease energy production. The pituitary gland is the vice president who relays those decisions. The thyroid is the company manager, sending out or holding back encouragement for energy production to each of the workers. And the mitochondria are those workers—and their activity has a huge impact, because there are *trillions* of them.

The scenario is actually a little more complicated, because various areas of your body can choose precisely when to make use of the thyroid hormones. It's as if your body was divided into different departments run by field-level managers, some of whom can decide whether the "speed up production" orders for the whole company are appropriate at that moment for that particular department. Overall, though, if your thyroid is churning out hormones, your cells will become more active.

Metabolism and Your Thyroid

The energy level set by your hypothalamus and enforced by your thyroid is called your *metabolism.* If you hear someone complaining that he's overweight because "I have a slow metabolism," he's actually saying that his thyroid is underactive. If that's truly the case, he should see a doctor (see Chapter 4). On the other hand, he may simply be eating too much and exercising too little (see Chapter 19).

As long as you're alive, your metabolism will never be set to zero. Even when you're doing nothing strenuous, your body needs to keep your heart beating, your lungs breathing, your brain processing information, and so on. A measure of this base level of activity is your *resting metabolic rate,* or *RMR,* which represents the minimum number of calories your body will burn up in 24 hours.

THYROIDIAN TIP

If you Google "resting metabolic rate," you'll find free online calculators that will approximate the number of calories your body burns in 24 hours based on such factors as your height, weight, age, and gender. For example, the RMR for a man is typically in the 1,600-2,000 calorie range, while the RMR for a woman is usually 1,200-1,400 calories.

Your RMR is responsible for burning up the vast majority of your calories—typically, 65-75 percent. And it's RMR that your thyroid is primarily designed to regulate.

Of course, you have some control over your body's energy management, too. When you choose to walk to work instead of drive, and to take the stairs instead of the elevator, you're sending messages to your brain to burn up more calories. Your hypothalamus will notice your demands for higher production and set in motion the sequence of events that causes your cells to turn stored fat into glucose, and then ATP.

Exercise and other physical activity typically burn up only 15-25 percent of your calories. (The other 10 percent is used up dealing with food.) However, intense exercise can also raise your RMR for hours afterward, burning additional calories indirectly. Further, if you exercise regularly you'll reduce fat and increase lean muscle, and *that* will raise your metabolism, and your RMR, to a perpetual new high. (To learn more, see Chapters 19 and 20.)

So while there's a lot of energy regulation going on inside your body that you don't directly control, you can opt for adjustments to your lifestyle to make this system accommodate your wants and needs … as long as your thyroid is healthy.

If your thyroid starts malfunctioning, however, it will typically throw off your RMR by a whopping 30-40 percent in either direction—roughly the equivalent of the number of calories you'd burn by running six miles a day. And a change in weight is only one of many problems you may experience, as we'll discuss later in this chapter.

The Iodine Connection

Your thyroid makes its hormones by combining two ingredients that you consume every day (probably without even realizing it). The first is *tyrosine*, which is an amino acid that's found in many high-protein foods such as milk, cheese, yogurt, soy, chicken, turkey, fish, pumpkin seeds, sesame seeds, and almonds. Unless you're on a special low-protein diet, you're likely to have plenty of tyrosine in your system.

The second is *iodine*. Your thyroid is unique in that it's the only gland that absorbs iodine; the rest of your body ignores this chemical. You require only a tiny amount of iodine daily—generally 150-300 micrograms (mcg)—and whatever iodine you consume quickly gets sucked into your thyroid. If you eat fresh vegetables grown from iodine-rich soil or eat seafood, you probably take in all the iodine you need without even trying.

If you don't eat much produce, though, or if you live far from a coastal area (and from iodine-rich oceans), you may have to devote some attention to iodine.

That's especially so because iodine has become less ubiquitous. For example, it used to be the norm for fast-food restaurants and makers of processed foods to use iodized salt, which is a simple and inexpensive source of iodine (containing 45-80 mcg of iodine per gram of salt). But in part due to concerns about these salt-heavy food producers overdosing customers on iodine, most of these companies have switched to regular salt—which means a frozen dinner may provide you a great deal of sodium but zero iodine.

Similarly, in the past iodine was used in most baked goods as a dough conditioner. Now bromides often take its place, so there's no way to know whether your bread and rolls contain iodine unless you ask your bakery.

Dairy products also used to be a major source, because dairy manufacturers used iodine as a sanitizer; but synthetic compounds are now sometimes employed instead, so you can't consistently count on dairy foods as iodine sources.

If you have reason to suspect you're lacking in iodine, there are still many cheap and readily available sources. They include vegetables grown in iodine-rich soil, iodized salt, sea salt, and multivitamins that include 50-100 mcg of iodine. You can also eat seafood, including seaweed, which has lots of natural iodine. Inexpensive and low-calorie options include the seaweeds *nori*, *wakame*, and *dulse* (see Chapter 3).

THYROID FACTOID

While iodine is plentiful in most industrialized countries, it isn't everywhere. Hundreds of millions of people live in areas with iodine-deficient soil, and worldwide this is the top cause of thyroid-related ills—including such tragic birth defects as cretinism. Happily, this situation is improving. The World Health Organization has worked to reduce iodine deficiency from impacting 30 percent of the world's population in 1990 to less than 15 percent today.

While too little iodine will create thyroid issues, too much iodine isn't good either. You should consume no more than 1,000 mcg daily, and preferably stay within the 150-300 mcg range.

The "T" Factor

Assuming you have enough tyrosine and iodine in your system, your thyroid makes its hormones in two basic steps. First, it induces a chemical process that converts tyrosine into *thyroglobulin*, which is a protein specifically designed to bind with iodine. Your thyroid then combines a thyroglobulin molecule with 1 to 4 iodine atoms. The number of atoms attached determines the type of thyroid hormone that results.

If your thyroid attaches four iodine atoms, the hormone *thyroxine* (also called *tetra-iodothyronine*) is produced. It's most commonly referred to as *T4* because it's made from a thyroglobulin molecule (T) combined with four iodine atoms (4). T4 comprises 80-90 percent of the hormones made by your thyroid.

T4 is a "storage" hormone. Instead of performing actions on your body, it's designed to circulate in your bloodstream, and be stored in your tissues, until thyroid hormones are needed by a particular area of your body.

When energy is called for, an enzyme named *deiodinase type 1* is used to strip off a single iodine atom from the outer ring of T4 molecules. Deiodinase type 1 is stored in your liver, kidneys, brain, pituitary gland, muscles, skin, and tissues, making it rapidly available to every area of your body.

Converting T4 to a thyroid hormone with three iodine atoms results in *tri-iodothyronine*, or *T3*. And it's T3 that actually does the work of powering up the mitochondria in your cells.

DEFINITION

T4 and **T3** are the most important of the four hormones produced by your thyroid. T4 is a storage hormone that circulates in your bloodstream, or resides in your tissues, until some area of your body needs energy. The T4 is then converted into T3; and the T3 enters cells and "recharges" them by powering up their mitochondria.

It may seem wasteful to create T4 just so it can be transformed into T3. But T4 remains potent for about eight days in your bloodstream and tissues, while T3 retains its power for only around 10 hours. T4 therefore gives each region of your body the flexibility of having a thyroid hormone constantly available, and then "activating" it via conversion to T3 whenever a quick energy boost is needed.

In addition to T3 being created via T4 conversion, your thyroid makes T3 directly, although in much smaller quantities than T4. Your thyroid's T4-to-T3 production ratio is roughly 10:1. (Put another way, around 10 percent of the hormones your thyroid produces are T3.)

No one is certain why your thyroid creates T3 along with T4; but it's become a source of heated controversy. If your thyroid is underperforming, most doctors will prescribe *Synthroid*, which is a synthetic version of T4. The theory is that since your body can convert T4 to T3, Synthroid's T4 is all you need. However, many thyroid experts argue that your thyroid must be producing both T4 and T3 for a good reason, and that your medication should therefore also be a mix of T4 and T3. That's backed up by real-world experience; as many as 1 out of 3 patients don't do well with T4 medication alone. As a result, an increasing number of doctors are prescribing a combination of Synthroid and *Cytomel* (which is synthetic T3); or *desiccated thyroid* such as *Nature-Throid* (which is a natural mix of T4 and T3 derived from the thyroid of pigs). To learn more and decide which option is best for you, see Chapters 3 and 8.

THYROIDIAN TIP

The enzyme deiodinase type 1 is made in part from the chemical *selenium*. If you happen to be low on selenium (which can be detected via blood tests), then your body won't be able to convert enough T4 to T3. The simplest solution is to eat a single Brazil nut daily, which provides around 80 mcg of selenium. You'll receive the rest of the 200 mcg of selenium you need without even trying from eating other nuts, whole grains, and/or seafood. Don't regularly eat more than one Brazil nut a day, though, or you'll end up overdosing. (You can also buy selenium in 200 mcg pill form, but consuming it via food is actually more effective … and more fun.)

While T4 and T3 comprise the vast majority of hormones your thyroid produces, they're not the whole story. Roughly 4 percent of these hormones are *T2* and *T1*. As you've probably guessed by now, T2, or *do-iodothyronine*, is made with two iodine atoms. Until recently, most doctors considered T2 to be useless. Some researchers didn't believe your thyroid would create something for no reason, however, so they took a closer look; and now preliminary studies indicate T2 plays a role in metabolism and burning fat. It may also help with T4-to-T3 conversion. *Mono-iodothyronine*, or *T1*, still has no known purpose so far. However, researchers are taking a close look at it, too.

T2 and T1 are especially relevant when considering treatment. The only prescription medication that includes all four types of thyroid hormone is desiccated thyroid. That means if your thyroid has entirely stopped working, or if your thyroid has been removed, desiccated thyroid is your only option for continuing to have a normal amount of T2 and T1 in your body. Your doctor may give you a hard time if you request desiccated thyroid, but the reasons she provides are likely to be historical ones that have been obsolete for decades; to learn more, see Chapter 3.

One other thyroid hormone you may hear about is *reverse T3*. This is created when a batch of T4 is no longer needed (e.g., after it has outlived its "expiration date" of potency, or when your bloodstream has too much T4). Just as your body creates T3 by stripping off an iodine atom from the outer ring of T4 molecules, it creates reverse T3 by stripping off an iodine atom from the inner ring of T4 molecules. The reverse T3 will then be flushed out of your body.

> **CRASH GLANDING**
>
> Some alternative medicine practitioners claim reverse T3 has special significance in diagnosing disease (see Chapter 3). However, to date the evidence doesn't support reverse T3 being notable as anything other than an efficient way for your body to dispose of T4.

When Thyroids Go Wrong

Your thyroid normally creates just the right amount of hormones for your body's current needs, keeping all your cells active and operating smoothly. If your thyroid becomes defective, though, you'll probably experience a bewildering set of disparate ailments because of the thyroid's pervasive impact on all parts of the body. (For details, see Chapter 2.)

The three diseases that most frequently affect the thyroid are *hypothyroidism*, *hyperthyroidism*, and *thyroid cancer*. There are also a number of diseases that are less common or affect the thyroid indirectly.

Hypothyroidism

If you're *hypothyroid*, your thyroid is underperforming— essentially, not making enough T4 and/or T3. This is by far the most common of all thyroid diseases, comprising over 80 percent of thyroid cases.

When your body doesn't have enough thyroid hormones, the mitochondria in your cells will reduce their conversion of glucose into ATP. The unused glucose will be stored in your body as fat, causing you to gain weight. You'll also start feeling increasingly tired as your energy supply winds down.

In addition, your body cutting down on the generation of new cells may cause your nails to grow dry and brittle, your skin to become rough and thin, and your hair to thin and fall out. At the same time, the lowered brain activity may make you confused, forgetful, and even dangerously depressed.

You can experience any of these symptoms, and/or dozens of others, because the "energy slowdown" caused by your underperforming thyroid will have different effects on different parts of your body.

Hypothyroidism is a complicated disease. With the help of this book, however, the chances are high that you'll be able to navigate the various difficulties and obtain treatment that resolves all your thyroid problems. To find out much more, see Chapters 5 through 9.

DEFINITION

Hypothyroidism is by far the most common of thyroid diseases. It's caused by your thyroid underproducing its hormones, which reduces your energy and impairs the function of cells throughout your body. This can result in numerous ailments, ranging from the relatively trivial (brittle nails) to the devastating (severe depression). Fortunately, once it's correctly diagnosed, hypothyroidism is highly treatable.

Hyperthyroidism

If you're *hyperthyroid*, your thyroid is overperforming—essentially, making too much T4 and/or T3. This accounts for roughly 15 percent of thyroid cases.

When your body has an overabundance of thyroid hormones, the mitochondria in your cells will turn glucose into ATP at a much faster pace than normal. Once the available glucose runs out, your body will start turning your fat cells into glucose to keep up with the mitochondria's demand for more fuel, causing you to lose weight. You might actually be happy about the latter. However, you'll also start feeling increasingly manic from the extra energy.

You may also feel exceptionally anxious, nervous, irritable, or "shaky," and experience panic attacks. In addition, your heart rate may increase to the point of pounding in your chest, which poses the risk of a heart attack.

Hyperthyroidism is a more dangerous disease than hypothyroidism, and it requires more complex treatment. However, in most cases it's thoroughly manageable. For details, see Chapters 10 through 12.

DEFINITION

Hyperthyroidism occurs when your thyroid overproduces its hormones, raising your body's energy level beyond healthy limits. The overstimulation can cause such ills as tremors, severe anxiety, and a dangerously rapid heartbeat. Hyperthyroidism is treatable, but often requires time and patience until you either become healthy again or go in the other direction and become hypothyroid (which is a much easier disease to manage).

Thyroid Cancer

The thyroid disease that causes the most terror is thyroid cancer. It's relatively rare, comprising about 1 percent of thyroid disease cases. It's on the rise, however, with an increasingly greater number of people being struck every year.

Cancer has a reputation of being deadly and untreatable. Fortunately, that usually doesn't apply to thyroid cancer, which is about as treatable as cancer gets. The most common thyroid cancers, *papillary* and *follicular*, have a cure rate of 97 percent. If you have thyroid cancer, your treatment will typically consist of surgically removing the thyroid, and then giving you a dose of radioactive iodine. Because your thyroid is the only part of your body that absorbs iodine, the iodine will be ignored by the rest of your body and enter only whatever thyroid cells remain post-surgery—including all the cancer cells—at which point the radiation will obliterate them.

For a detailed description of diagnosing and dealing with thyroid cancer, see Chapter 13.

Other Thyroid-Related Problems

There are a number of other things that can go wrong in your body that either affect your thyroid or are affected by your thyroid.

For example, your thyroid does its job in partnership with your *adrenal glands*, which facilitate the conversion of T4 to T3, and also allow T3 to enter cell membranes and access mitochondria. If your adrenals malfunction, lab tests will still show your thyroid to be working perfectly … because it is. But since your thyroid hormones are being blocked from doing their work, you'll nonetheless be hypothyroid. To learn more about this subtle problem, see Chapter 14.

Other ailments that are in some way connected to your thyroid include parathyroid disease, thyroiditis, thyroid eye disease, and MEN syndrome. For details, see Chapter 15.

Two special problem areas resulting from thyroid disease that often don't get enough attention are mental and emotional disorders, and women's issues such as PMS, fertility, and menopause. These are covered in Chapters 16 and 17.

Why Thyroids Go Wrong

Thyroid disease is as old as mankind. In ancient times its primary cause was a lack of iodine. That's no longer a serious issue in industrialized countries such as the United States, but a modern problem has taken its place: environmental toxins.

Your thyroid is extraordinarily effective at drawing in and storing iodine. That's normally a good thing. However, there are a number of substances that are chemically similar to iodine, such as mercury and perchlorate. Small amounts of such chemicals may find their way into your body via processed foods, pesticides on produce, poor quality water, etc. If your thyroid mistakes them for iodine, it'll suck them up and store them, too.

Over time, the amount of unhealthy chemicals that accumulate in your thyroid can become so significant that they'll trigger your body's immune system. Your body will designate them as foreign invaders, and create antibodies to attack them and flush them out of your system. Unfortunately, the antibodies will often mistake your thyroid as an accomplice of the toxins (which, in a way, it is) and also attack your thyroid cells.

This is called an *autoimmune* response; and it's responsible for the vast majority of both hypothyroidism and hyperthyroidism. Experts believe this is why thyroid disease is so prevalent. Every year increasingly more chemicals are being pumped into both the environment and our food supply; and the older you get, the more toxins will accumulate in your thyroid.

That said, there are a number of things you can do to improve your chances of avoiding or mitigating thyroid disease. For numerous tips on how to avoid toxins, eat healthy, and live healthy, see Chapters 18 through 22.

One other problem in our modern age is low-level radiation, which is believed to be the primary cause of thyroid cancer (see Chapter 13). Complicating matters is that radiation is among the treatments for hyperthyroidism. For the pros and cons of pursuing this treatment, see Chapter 12.

The Least You Need to Know

- Thyroid disease has become an epidemic in the United States, striking 1 in 10 Americans.
- Your thyroid regulates the energy level of every cell in your body.
- Thyroid hormones are made from iodine, which you can get from eating iodized salt, seafood, and/or fresh vegetables.
- T4 is a "storage" hormone that your body converts to T3 when you need energy.
- The primary causes of thyroid disease in industrialized countries such as the United States are environmental toxins and low-level radiation.

Sorting Through Symptoms

In This Chapter

- Identifying thyroid disease symptoms
- Weight and energy changes
- Mental and sexual issues
- Hair, nail, and skin problems
- Testing your suspicions

Thyroid disease is often hard to identify because it can create any of dozens of wildly varying symptoms, ranging from weight change to insomnia to brittle nails to mood swings. Even superb doctors who don't happen to be experts in this area can fail to realize when a problem is being caused by an ailing thyroid.

The good news is we're here to help. In this chapter, we'll guide you through the most common symptoms of thyroid disease, complete with real-life stories about patients who had one or more of these issues and thoroughly overcame them with inexpensive thyroid medication.

Once you're done reading, you'll have a checklist of symptoms you can take to your doctor for testing, diagnosis, and possible treatment.

Hearing Your Thyroid's Messages

As explained in Chapter 1, your thyroid regulates the energy levels of your body by producing hormones that make your cells increase or decrease their activity. Because these hormones affect organs, tissues, and cells throughout your body, if your thyroid starts malfunctioning you may experience myriad problems stemming from your brain, your colon, your skin, your neck … the possibilities are overwhelming.

Some symptoms may be obvious, such as trouble swallowing or eye pain. Others may be so subtle—such as feeling irritable or becoming forgetful—that you're unlikely to immediately recognize them as the results of an illness.

Diagnosing thyroid disease is tricky for doctors. Different patients can have completely different symptoms, combinations of symptoms, and severity of symptoms, all stemming from an off-kilter thyroid.

While most thyroid-related issues aren't immediately serious, they can become dangerous over time. And either way, they have a significant negative impact on quality of life. There are millions of people who suffer from debilitating problems simply because neither they nor their doctors have recognized the root cause as a defective thyroid. It's a tragedy, because thyroid disease is usually easy to treat … but not until it's been identified.

For example, I had a patient we'll call Margaret (the names of all patients mentioned in this book have been changed to protect their privacy) who'd been seeing me as her general practitioner for several years. During a routine check-up I asked Margaret if she was sleeping well, and she casually replied, "Actually, I've been having insomnia." I noticed she looked a little too thin, so I checked her weight; it was down 14 pounds from the previous year. Margaret told me she wasn't dieting: "I just haven't been as hungry lately, no big deal." I noticed she was sweating even though the room was cool, and her resting heart rate was a rapid 100 beats per minute. If I weren't an expert on thyroid symptoms, I might have prescribed sleeping pills instead of putting the pieces together. Instead, I tested Margaret and, as I suspected, she was suffering from hyperthyroidism. Medication soon eliminated all the problems and restored Margaret to a happy life.

Too often we rationalize changes in our bodies, altering our perception of what's normal rather than acknowledging that there's something wrong.

This chapter will empower you to listen to your body when it's saying your thyroid isn't doing its job.

Thyroid Disease Symptoms Checklist

Because thyroid hormones affect every cell, in theory an ailing thyroid can result in any of hundreds of different symptoms. In general, though, certain symptoms are more likely to occur than others. These frequent clues to thyroid malfunction appear in the checklist that follows.

Take a few minutes to go over the list and check off any symptom that applies to you. If you aren't sure whether you have a particular symptom, find the description of it later in this chapter and use the additional information to make your decision.

Thyroid Disease Symptoms Checklist

- ❏ Gaining weight for no apparent reason
- ❏ Losing weight for no apparent reason
- ❏ Frequent exhaustion
- ❏ Sluggishness
- ❏ Nervousness
- ❏ Anxiety
- ❏ Irritability
- ❏ Feeling "shaky"
- ❏ Slowed thinking
- ❏ Memory problems
- ❏ Depression
- ❏ Lowered interest in sex
- ❏ Excessive interest in sex
- ❏ Menstrual problems
- ❏ Infertility
- ❏ Insomnia
- ❏ Constipation
- ❏ Unusually frequent bowel movements
- ❏ Hair loss
- ❏ Thinning or dry hair
- ❏ Dry, brittle nails
- ❏ Rough, itchy, and/or thinning skin

❑ Acne

❑ Puffy skin

❑ Cold skin

❑ Feeling unusually cold

❑ Sweating too little or too much

❑ Numbness or tingling in the hands and feet

❑ Rapidly beating heart

❑ Weak muscles

❑ Painful and/or enlarged eyes

❑ Hoarse voice

❑ Enlarged neck

If you have six or more of these common symptoms, there's a strong chance your thyroid is ailing. Get your thyroid checked out—typically via blood tests for TSH, free T4, free T3, and antibodies—as soon as possible.

If you have two to five of these symptoms, that's still reason enough to get your thyroid tested. Either the results will be positive, putting you on the path to treatment, or negative, which will inform your doctor to explore other potential problem sources. (Before accepting a negative result, though, see Chapter 7.)

But even if you have only one of these symptoms and your doctor isn't providing a satisfying explanation for its cause, you should seriously consider getting tested. That's doubly true if you're a woman who's 30-50 years old, as that's the gender and age range most often struck by hypothyroidism.

The checklist is by no means comprehensive; you can definitely experience other symptoms. However, the odds are that along with the unlisted symptoms you'll have at least a few of the ones on the checklist. If you're successfully treated for thyroid disease, you'll soon experience improvement regarding *all* your thyroid-related symptoms.

THYROIDIAN TIP

Virtually any symptom on the checklist can be caused by something beyond a faulty thyroid. Therefore, ask your doctor to give you a full physical, and to explore other potential causes *in addition* to the thyroid testing. Even if your symptoms turn out to be entirely thyroid-related, that doesn't mean the search for causes should end. For example, if you have an autoimmune thyroid disease, it might have developed from toxins in your system. Eliminating such toxins (by changing your water supply, switching to organic food, etc.) could result in your eventually not needing thyroid medication … and lead to overall better health.

The rest of this chapter describes common thyroid-related symptoms in more depth, then concludes with some advice about testing.

Weight and Energy Symptoms

By far the most well-known symptoms of an ailing thyroid are weight gain and low energy (for hypothyroidism), or weight loss and excessive energy (for hyperthyroidism). Both issues are related to your metabolism, which your thyroid can inadvertently set to operate too slowly or too quickly.

Gaining or Losing Weight

Your thyroid controls your resting metabolic rate (RMR), which is the rate at which your body burns calories when at rest. To better understand this concept, think of your body as a car that never shuts off. When the car is moving, it burns up gasoline at a higher rate. But even when it's just idling, it's burning up a significant amount of fuel.

If you're like most people, you probably burn 1,300-2,000 calories daily from your resting metabolic rate (and another 300-700 calories from activities). So if an off-kilter thyroid changes your RMR by even just a third, it has an enormous impact on your body's calorie consumption.

If your thyroid suddenly starts underproducing hormones, your body's "idle" rate will go down, making you burn fewer calories per hour. This will cause you to gain weight … possibly a lot of weight. Even if you eat less and exercise more, it probably won't be enough to compensate for your lowered metabolism.

For example, Elizabeth was convinced her thyroid was off because she was struggling so hard with her weight. Noticing she was 5'9" and weighed 117 pounds, at first I thought she had a body image problem. Then she explained she thought her current weight was fine, but she was taking extreme measures to maintain it. Six days a week Elizabeth got up at 4:00 A.M., ran 10 miles, and then spent another 30-45 minutes at the gym before going to work. And her diet consisted primarily of fruits and vegetables, never exceeding 900 calories a day! That's all I needed to hear to be convinced testing was called for; and it turned out Elizabeth was indeed suffering from hypothyroidism. Once we got her on medication, she was able to maintain her weight eating 1,400-1,600 calories and no more than an hour of exercise daily.

Alternatively, if your thyroid suddenly starts overproducing hormones, your body's "idle" rate will go up, making you burn more calories per hour. This will cause you to lose weight. If you've been overweight, that'll be good news … temporarily. But over time, you'll become dangerously thin.

In either case, thyroid treatment will return your metabolism to normal.

THYROIDIAN TIP

Just because you gain weight doesn't mean you have a thyroid or metabolism problem. If you tend to eat a lot and not exercise, a weight gain is to be expected. However, if you've maintained a steady weight, and then suddenly start gaining with no change in your diet or exercise habits, then thyroid testing is called for.

Sluggishness or Exhaustion

If you're a workaholic getting by on six hours of sleep a day, it's no surprise you feel exhausted. But if you have a reasonable schedule and normal sleep habits, and for no apparent reason suddenly feel burned out daily, something's wrong.

See if any of the following statements ring a bell:

- You're pushing yourself just to get through the day.

- Activities you used to love are such a strain that you've stopped enjoying them.

- You've stopped exercising, socializing, etc., because you can't spare the energy.

- You crash in the afternoon, wanting to do nothing but sleep.

- When you get home from work, you feel so dead tired that all you can do is sleep.

If any item on this list resonates, and there's no clear cause for the problem, seeing a doctor and getting tested for hypothyroidism is a good idea.

Mental Symptoms

It's obvious an ailing thyroid can cause physical problems. But what many people—including a fair number of doctors—don't realize is the profound effect the thyroid has on your mental health. Your brain is one of the organs most affected by thyroid hormones. When that supply is thrown off-balance, your thoughts and emotions may soon follow.

The next three sections cover thyroid-related mental issues that can wreak havoc on the quality of your life until they're identified and treated.

Depression and Anxiety

If you're experiencing depression, anxiety, or moodiness, you may find friends disregarding these feelings as being "just in your mind." You may even rationalize them yourself as being tied to outside circumstances, such as stress at work. (In the past our ancestors blamed problems on hexes; in our modern age we blame them on stress.)

But if your mental difficulties are ongoing, and if you have other thyroid-related symptoms (fatigue, weight change, hair loss, etc.) along with them, you shouldn't hesitate to get tested. In fact, even if you have no other symptoms but you can't identify a cause for the problem, a thyroid test is worth doing.

For example, Brittany came to see me for anxiety. She said it was caused by her boss feeling nothing she did was good enough—but upon questioning her, I learned Brittany's performance evaluations were always positive and she received a raise after every review. Clearly there was something else going on. As we talked more, I learned Brittany was just as anxious about her relationships with friends, her personal safety, and various other areas of her life. Her anxiety actually had nothing to do with work or stress.

Brittany had undergone talk therapy with an experienced psychologist, and had also tried anti-anxiety medication. None of it helped. The psychiatrist referred her to me to see if there was a possible physical cause. Brittany had no other symptoms, but since she'd reached a dead end, I saw no harm in testing her thyroid as part of a blood evaluation.

To my surprise, the lab tests were positive. It's unusual for thyroid disease to manifest with just one symptom; but as Brittany's case demonstrates, every now and then it happens. And if I hadn't ordered that $50 test, Brittany might have struggled with anxiety for years, wrecking her life.

Instead, over the course of four months I gently raised Brittany's dose of thyroid medication, and frequently checked her blood until her levels normalized. Even with no therapy or other medication, the intrusive thoughts that disrupted her days virtually disappeared. On the rare occasion when Brittany felt anxious, she was able to make the discomfort go away simply by exercising.

Even worse than anxiety is depression, which is one of the most devastating diseases for one's quality of life. In the words of a patient: "The really odd part about this is there's nothing upsetting or unusual going on in my life. And yet I notice my mood has significantly shifted. I don't have any interest in things I did before, I have to force myself to do much of anything, and I'm not enjoying anything."

If you have depression along with other thyroid-related symptoms, get tested. That said, there have been studies in which patients didn't test positive for thyroid disease but weren't responding to antidepressants, so T3 (in the form of Cytomel) was added to the mix of meds to see if it would help regardless. In the majority of cases, it did. No data exists on whether doctors misinterpreted the lab tests (see Chapter 7) and the patients really had thyroid problems after all. At any rate, using T3 as a supplement to antidepressants is becoming increasingly common.

THYROIDIAN TIP

If your doctor is prescribing Cytomel as a supplement to other medication, make sure he's monitoring your thyroid blood levels via TSH, free T4, and free T3 tests. Otherwise you could end up with too much T3 in your system and start experiencing hyperthyroid symptoms.

Fogginess and/or Forgetfulness

Roughly 20 percent of the calories burned up during your resting metabolic state are used by your brain. If your thyroid hormones decrease, they'll set your brain to be less active and fire up less frequently. As a result, your thinking may slow down, leading you to feel foggy and unfocused.

You may also have trouble remembering even simple things like the names of people you know, where you put your keys, the reason you're standing in your closet ....

There are other possible causes of these symptoms. But if they occur along with fatigue, depression, etc., have your thyroid checked.

Nervousness and/or Irritability

Nervousness, irritability, and shakiness are typically thought of as hyperthyroid symptoms—that is, the results of your body being too revved up. And, in fact, they are. But they can *also* be evidence of hypothyroidism—particularly if they're accompanied by anxiety.

Either way, if you have such symptoms and there's no other clear cause, get tested. The results will tell you precisely what's going on.

Having Trouble Sleeping

When your thyroid is malfunctioning, your mind may fill with disjointed thoughts. This can result in your having trouble falling asleep as your mind sorts through all the things you experienced that day, and all the things you plan to do the next day. Alternatively, you may fall asleep normally, but then wake up soon afterward because your brain is having trouble doing its normal nighttime job of processing information.

There's also some interplay between thyroid-related symptoms. For example, if you're suffering from fatigue, it could cause insomnia because you need to get "played out" to properly unwind and sleep at night. That can't happen if you're too tired to be active.

There are so many potential causes for a sleep disorder that this symptom by itself shouldn't make you think "thyroid." But it's definitely notable when combined with other thyroid-related symptoms.

Sex and Fertility Symptoms

Thyroid hormones directly affect the gonads, and so influence ovary and testicle functioning. This can impact menstruation, fertility, and sexual feelings.

For example, if you're a woman with an underperforming thyroid, your ovaries may do a poor job of synthesizing estrogen and progesterone, causing your menstrual cycles to become irregular. In more severe cases, it may also cause dysfunctional heavy bleeding, and make the ovarian lining inadequate for proper fertilization. The latter can cause infertility, or lead to a miscarriage.

It's also quite common for hypothyroidism to affect sexual desire—when your thyroid becomes underactive, your libido often will, too. That's in part because of the connection between thyroid hormones and your sexual organs. In addition, when your metabolism slows down, you're likely to feel less energetic and enthusiastic about *everything* … including sex.

For example, my patient Sandra had a very active sex life with her husband for the first three years of marriage; her girlfriends referred to them as "the bunnies." But over the next two years, she lost interest. "It's gotten so bad," she told me, "that I've begun making secret marks on the calendar to remind me to initiate sex at least a few times a month. Otherwise it wouldn't even occur to me."

Sandra wanted to try testosterone therapy. I told her that we first needed to run tests to determine the root cause of the problem. To be thorough, I included a thyroid test; and to my surprise, even though Sandra had no other thyroid-related symptoms, she tested positive for advanced hypothyroidism. As mentioned previously, it's unusual for one thyroid symptom to appear in isolation—but it can definitely happen.

After several months of treatment, I received a "thank you" card from a man I didn't know. It had nothing on it but an illustration of two rabbits lounging by a river. I checked the last name against my patient records … and realized it was from Sandra's husband.

Irregularity Symptoms

Your small intestine and colon form a very long tube lined by rings. Think about "the wave" crowds do at sports stadiums. That's sort of what happens in this tube; the first ring fires, and then the next ring, and so on, coaxing undigested material through your body. This process is called *peristalsis*, and its intensity is regulated by thyroid hormones.

If you're hypothyroid, peristalsis will be sluggish. As a result, you may experience constipation. In addition, you may absorb more calories, because food is lingering longer in your long intestine and colon—which means you'll gain weight even faster from eating exactly the same amount of food as usual. Further, you risk being exposed to more toxins, because bad chemicals that normally would be flushed out of your system quickly are instead sticking around.

Conversely, if you're hyperthyroid, peristalsis is sped up. This can lead to increased bowel movements and/or loose stools. In addition, the undigested food racing through your body doesn't allow enough time for calories to be absorbed adequately. This is a major reason for losing weight under hyperthyroidism.

Occasional constipation and excessive bowel movements aren't unusual. But if the problem is ongoing, and no other cause is evident, your thyroid is worth considering as the culprit.

Hair, Skin, and Nail Symptoms

When you have hypothyroidism, your body is forced to make a choice. With limited resources to call upon, it focuses energy on vital functions such as keeping you breathing, while diverting energy from nonessentials … which include keeping your hair thick and full, skin soft and supple, and nails strong and healthy.

The latter are structural parts of your body. Hypothyroidism won't make them break down any quicker; but it may greatly slow down the rebuilding process, leading to eventual degeneration. It's like a city neglecting its infrastructure. Everything will keep running, but over time it'll look increasingly awful.

Hair That's Thin or Falling Out

If your hair becomes dry or thin, that's notable for thyroid concerns only in combination with other thyroid-related symptoms.

If you're losing hair, though, the details become meaningful. When caused by hypothyroidism, hair loss won't be patchy or localized, but instead diffuse, even, and non-patterned. And it will typically include the full length of the shafts and follicles, as opposed to hair merely breaking off.

Most importantly, the hair loss will happen at a substantially greater rate than what you were used to when your thyroid was normal.

THYROID FACTOID

Your head has around 100,000 hairs. So even if you start losing hair due to hypothyroidism, it will take years before you become bald—and because you're reading this book, you'll be on thyroid medication long before that happens.

Even better news is that if you're treated within two years, the chances are all the hair you lost will grow back.

Rough, Itchy, and/or Thinning Skin

Your skin's cells have a very high rate of turnover; they're continually flaking off and being replaced. When your body's repair rate slows down, though, your skin will become rough, calloused, itchy, and/or thin—especially on your fingertips, hands, upper arms, and feet.

Acne

When your body's energy decreases, the reduced maintenance of your skin can cause fatty acids and other wastes to build up and clog your pores. This makes your skin more vulnerable to bacterial infection, and may lead to various forms of acne such as pimples, boils, whiteheads, and blackheads … even if you're long past the teen years usually associated with acne.

Puffy and/or Cold Skin

Hypothyroidism causes a fluid called mucin to build up right below the skin. This results in a puffy appearance.

THYROID FACTOID

Centuries ago doctors didn't understand the role of the thyroid in disease, but they noticed when patients came in with swelling from mucin buildup so severe it could be spotted from across the room. In 1877 the condition was named *myxedema;* and to this day you may see the term myxedema used interchangeably with hypothyroidism.

Further, because your metabolism slows down, there's less energy available to generate heat. This can make you feel cold, as well as lower your skin's resistance to cold. For example, you may find yourself bringing a sweater along wherever you go because you expect to feel colder than anyone else in the room. The feeling of cold tends to be specially prominent in the feet and hands; so you may also suddenly find yourself wearing heavy socks to bed, or wearing gloves when you've never needed to before.

Dry, Brittle Nails

There are a number of ways your nails may become dry, lined, brittle, and break easily. For example, if you switch to a restrictive diet, or if you develop digestive problems, your nails will be affected by a decrease in minerals such as zinc, and by a decrease in protein. But if nothing's changed in your life, your nails going downhill may indicate a thyroid issue.

Other Symptoms

As mentioned previously, a malfunctioning thyroid can lead to scores of different problems. The next six sections cover some of the most common ones that don't fit neatly into any category.

Racing Heart

One of the most frequent symptoms of hyperthyroidism is a rapidly beating heart. In fact, if you start taking thyroid medication, a good doctor will ask you to pay attention to ongoing heart palpitations, because that's the most obvious sign your thyroid levels are getting too high and you need to scale back on the meds (in which case you should contact your doctor about getting retested ASAP).

In the earliest stages of hyperthyroidism you might not notice your heart beating more quickly during the day, when you have lots of distractions, but you may become aware of it at night as you lay quietly in bed. As the disease progresses, your increased heartbeat will become more pronounced. At that point you shouldn't think twice about seeing a doctor.

THYROIDIAN TIP

If you're hyperthyroid, or suspect you are, avoid exercise until you've been fully treated. Normally exercise will take you from a resting heart rate of around 70 beats per second to 130 bps; but if your resting heart rate is abnormally rapid, exercise could raise it to a dangerously high level of 170-200 bps. And much worse, once your rate goes up that high, it might *stay* there even after you've finished your session. That's a risk not worth taking. Instead, skip working out until you're okay again.

Numb or Tingling Hands and Feet

Your thyroid regulates the rate at which your nerves conduct signals through your body.

If you're hypothyroid, your nerves may start conducting signals with less energy. This will slow down your reflexes, and may also cause sporadic numbness, especially in your hands and feet.

Conversely, if you're hyperthyroid, your nerves may relay signals with excessive energy. This can result in exaggerated reflexes, tremors, and/or sporadic tingling or pain, particularly in your hands and feet.

Weak Muscles

One of the paradoxes of thyroid disease is that certain conditions can be caused by both too little and too much thyroid hormones. And a prime example is weakened muscles.

If you're hypothyroid, your muscles are being told to reduce their activity. Because the body has a "use it or lose it" policy, over time this will sap their strength.

If you're hyperthyroid, your muscles are being told to get super-active; but at the same time you aren't absorbing the nutrients you need to nourish them.

So while the reasons are different, both conditions can produce the same symptom.

Irregular Sweating

Your sweat glands are regulated by thyroid hormones. As a result, if your thyroid is underactive, you may suddenly find yourself barely sweating under conditions in which you'd normally be pouring buckets. Conversely, if your thyroid is overactive, you may be sweating gallons for no apparent reason.

The areas of your body most affected are typically your underarms, hands, and back of your head. For example, if you normally go to the gym and sweat a ton under your arms, you could suddenly find your shirt is virtually dry after a workout. This makes it tougher for your body to expel heat and can make exercising uncomfortable. If this keeps happening and nothing else has changed, get tested.

Painful and/or Enlarged Eyes

Your eyes are vulnerable to a hyperthyroid state called *Graves' disease*. This condition spawns antibodies that may attack the fat and muscles near your eyes. This can make you sensitive to light; feel a painful dryness or grittiness in your eyes; or experience double vision. Even worse, as the disease progresses it can make your eyes protrude, creating a "bug-eyed" look. But if you're diagnosed during the early stages, an experienced doctor can treat you to keep that from happening.

Enlarged Neck and/or Hoarse Voice

There are a couple of ways your thyroid can grow so large that it affects your neck and/or your voice. When your pituitary gland senses your thyroid hormone levels are low, it tells your thyroid to grow new cells to get production back on track. That's normally a good thing. But if your thyroid develops a problem and substantially underachieves, your pituitary gland will respond by telling your thyroid to grow a lot larger than is good for you. In this case, one or more growths from your thyroid (called *goiters*) may get so big that they create a noticeable bulge in your neck. Further, they may put pressure on your nearby larynx, or *voice box*, causing your voice to sound hoarser. They could even make you have trouble swallowing.

Alternatively, a thyroid can develop smaller bumps, called *nodules*. Sometimes these nodules do no harm; but sometimes they're indications of thyroid cancer (see Chapter 13). As nodules continue growing, they're eventually visible as small bulges in the neck.

If you see or feel anything growing in your neck, see a doctor without delay. It'll probably be very treatable; but the sooner you're diagnosed, the better.

When in Doubt, Get Tested

If you've read through this chapter, you may now be feeling as if every ailment under the sun is caused by a faulty thyroid. Naturally, that's not the case. For example, most people who have weight problems simply eat too much and exercise too little. And most people who are fatigued just aren't giving their bodies enough rest and loving care.

But the chances are 10-20 percent of them really are suffering from thyroid disease. As explained in Chapter 1, thyroid disease has become an epidemic. Since thyroid blood tests are quick, easy, and relatively inexpensive, if you have a reasonable suspicion that your thyroid is malfunctioning, it's wise to err on the side of caution and get yourself tested.

If you don't have health insurance and are hesitant to see a doctor based on just a guess, you can perform preliminary blood tests yourself by drawing a blood sample at home and mailing it to a nationally certified lab. To find recommended companies that provide this service, visit this book's website at CIGThyroid.com. After your lab results arrive—typically within two weeks—you can use Chapter 7 (for hypothyroidism) or Chapter 11 (for hyperthyroidism) to interpret them.

If the numbers indicate a thyroid problem, get yourself insured and then go see a doctor for formal testing, diagnosis, and possible treatment. Beyond thyroid testing, a good doctor will perform a thorough check to identify other problems that might be causing your symptoms instead of—or in addition to—any thyroid issues. For advice on finding and selecting a physician, see Chapter 4.

The Least You Need to Know

- Seemingly unrelated symptoms can all be caused by thyroid disease.
- Symptoms can involve your weight, energy, thinking, mood, sex drive, heart, hair, nails, skin, and more.
- If you have even one thyroid-related symptom, get tested.
- Ask your doctor to test your thyroid *in addition* to other tests, not instead of them.

Thyroid Controversies

In This Chapter

- Avoiding bad practices
- Comparing synthetic and natural medications
- Comparing brand name and generic medications
- Avoiding unsafe remedies

If you research thyroid disease online or skim through other thyroid books, you'll quickly be struck by the wildly different theories competing for your attention. Some will scream that mainstream doctors can't be trusted. Others will claim that alternative doctors are quacks. Some will declare that taking synthetic medication is insane. Others will tell you natural medication is unreliable. Further, each side makes an argument that, at first blush, sounds convincing.

These battling schools of thought can be terribly confusing even to experienced doctors, let alone a patient just starting to learn about the thyroid. This chapter will therefore gently guide you through the most common thyroid controversies you're likely to encounter as you explore potential physicians, talk to friends, and cruise the web.

Why the Thyroid Breeds Controversy

Few other medical problems inspire as much heated debate as thyroid disease. Part of the reason is the ubiquitous nature of the thyroid, which behaves like your body's thermostat, controlling how much or how little energy you receive. This affects dozens of functions throughout your system, ranging from how quickly you lose weight to how much you want sex to how happy you are. All this can make the thyroid appear to have mysterious and magical powers … and that mystical aura tends to attract eccentrics and quacks.

Further, the wide range and subtlety of thyroid problems can make them difficult to diagnose. There aren't many disease states whose very existence is debatable, and the frustration this creates for patients naturally leads to strong feelings and passionately expressed opinions.

There are also genuine issues involved. Many mainstream doctors have fallen into bad habits, such as focusing on blood tests to the exclusion of symptoms, relying on health ranges suggested by labs rather than by thyroid experts, and prescribing only high-priced synthetic medications when inexpensive traditional drugs often do a better job.

At the same time, there are alternative doctors who stray from sound scientific practices, or even common sense, championing approaches that pose serious risks to their patients.

Another reason for the heat is an evolution in the doctor-patient relationship. It used to be that your doctor told you what to do and you did it, no questions asked. Many modern patients aren't satisfied with such a one-sided arrangement; they want to actively participate in their diagnosis and treatment. And when it comes to the often subtle symptoms of thyroid disease, that's absolutely appropriate.

What's unfortunate is that the discussion is so frequently framed as an "us against them" battle. There are extremely positive aspects to the strategies of both mainstream and alternative thyroid doctors, to the views of both doctors and patient advocates, and so on. People tend to get in trouble when they cut themselves off from the perspectives of others and become tunnel-visioned.

The key to success for a good thyroid doctor is having a balanced approach. And that's the attitude you should take with each controversy: a healthy mix of openness and skepticism.

THROAT QUOTE

Keep an open mind, but don't let your brain fall out.

—Anonymous

Broda Barnes and Basal Temperature

One of the champions in the history of thyroid disease is Dr. Broda Barnes. Barnes was a prominent voice in correctly declaring hypothyroidism as a vastly underdiagnosed illness. He also pointed out that doctors fail their patients if they focus so much on lab test results that they neglect paying close attention to patient symptoms. And he was an advocate for desiccated thyroid medication at a time when this important option was in danger of being wiped out.

In addition, Barnes and his co-author Lawrence Galton wrote the seminal 1976 book *Hypothyroidism: The Unsuspected Illness,* an exceptionally readable and compelling description of thyroid disease as Barnes understood it.

Barnes did fine work for his time; and his charismatic advocacy for a more organic approach to thyroid disease has won him followers who continue to use his methods. However, science has progressed since the days when Barnes practiced medicine. Certain techniques that he advocated 50 years ago simply aren't relevant in the twenty-first century.

Most prominently, Barnes advocated a diagnostic technique called the basal temperature test. This involved a patient placing a thermometer in his armpit for 10 minutes right after waking up. The reasoning was that a slowed metabolism results in a lower body temperature, and so a temperature of 97.8°F or below was evidence of hypothyroidism.

There are problems with this technique, though. Small variations in how a patient performs the test can create substantial differences in the result. There are other factors that can affect body temperature. And some temperatures Barnes considered evidence of a problem are now known to be normal for many patients.

Barnes developed the basal temperature test because the lab tests available in his time were woefully inadequate. Since then, however, medical science had made enormous progress. Labs can now process a small sample of your blood and provide remarkably precise and accurate information about how well or poorly your thyroid is performing.

So if you run across anyone who claims lab tests are useless and the only proper tool for diagnosing your thyroid's condition is the basal temperature test, that person is living in the past.

Along the same lines, if you learn a doctor you're considering bases her practice on the techniques of Barnes, seek a different doctor who has the same spirit of caring and attention to symptoms as Barnes did, but is also committed to using modern medical tools.

Wilson's Syndrome

In the late 1980s, E. Denis Wilson, a Florida doctor, declared he'd discovered a disease that was "the most common of all chronic ailments and probably takes a greater toll on society than any other medical condition." Rather immodestly, he termed it *Wilson's syndrome*. (You may also hear it called *Wilson's temperature syndrome* or *Wilson's thyroid syndrome*.) The symptoms described by Wilson echo those caused by thyroid disease—fatigue, hair loss, depression, etc. However, Wilson claimed standard thyroid tests often don't pick up Wilson's Syndrome because it's caused by an excess of reverse T3.

More specifically, when your thyroid produces hormones, the bulk of it is T4. The T4 can't be used by your body as is, however; so when your body is ready for increased energy, it removes an iodine atom, converting the T4 to useable T3. That's not the whole story, though. Your thyroid will typically produce more T4 than you need, and the T4 will remain in your system until it's degraded by losing an iodine atom. So what your body does with excess T4 is remove a different iodine atom, turning it into reverse T3. Reverse T3 is inactive and will simply be flushed out of your system.

Doctors don't normally test for reverse T3 because it's considered meaningless information, but Wilson based an entire theory of disease on reverse T3. Who's right? According to most reputable experts, not Wilson.

THYROID FACTOID

Back when Wilson first came out with his theory, I decided to check it out by having my lab run reverse T3 tests on over 100 of my patients along with their standard tests. There was no evidence of elevated reverse T3 for any of my patients; the reverse T3 data proved to be random noise. In fairness, Wilson claims the problem can take place within cells, which wouldn't show up on blood tests. (In place of lab tests, Wilson relies on the Broda Barnes basal temperature test described in the previous section.) But if there's no hard evidence of a claim, how seriously can you take it?

Nonetheless, Wilson devised an elaborate treatment for his syndrome that involves escalating and decreasing doses of compounded time-released T3. For example, a dose might start at 5 micrograms and work its way up to 100 mcg in the course of a week, and then work its way back down again. The appeal of the process is that it's supposed to permanently cure all symptoms.

But aside from there being no reason to believe the treatment does any good, it's dangerous. In fact, one of Wilson's own patients died of heart failure after taking large amounts of thyroid hormones. In 1992, the Florida Board of Medicine suspended Wilson's license to practice. However, Wilson continues to write, lecture, and give seminars, and other doctors have taken up his ideas.

Guy Abraham's Iodine Project

According to such universally respected organizations as the USDA and the World Health Organization, an adult should consume around 150-300 mcg of iodine per day, and shouldn't exceed 1,000 mcg—that's 1 *milligram*—of iodine daily.

Around two decades ago, however, Dr. Guy Abraham ran across some studies suggesting that megadoses of iodine could stop fibrocystic breast disease. These papers were recommending 5-20 milligrams a day—as much as 20 times what the USDA considers the maximum safe dosage. Abraham extrapolated from this that megadoses of iodine would be good for everyone … and especially patients with thyroid problems.

He blamed recommendations for 150-300 mcg per day on "iodophobia," a term he made up that refers to an irrational fear of iodine. According to Abraham, the right way to determine your appropriate iodine dosage is by swallowing a 50 milligram tablet of his own product Iodoral and then collecting your urine over the next 24 hours for testing. The rationale is that whatever iodine you don't pee out in a day is iodine your body must have needed.

After your first Iodoral experience, you're placed on a daily dose of it, and periodically retested. Your iodine doses keep increasing until you're peeing out more than you're taking in. The problem with this process is that your body doesn't actually eliminate toxins with perfect efficiency (and at such high dosages, the iodine is indeed a toxin). It's a bit like giving you a high dose of mercury and then saying, "If you didn't pee it all out after a day, your body must be craving more mercury."

When your iodine intake abruptly increases, it can actually take months for your body to adjust and learn to expel the excess amounts in your urine. Meanwhile, overloading your thyroid with iodine can cause it to shut down, creating a state of hypothyroidism. Over time, it can also increase the risk of developing goiters, Graves' disease, Hashimoto's disease, or even thyroid cancer.

Nonetheless, a significant number of alternative medicine practitioners champion Abraham's theories.

Desiccated vs. Synthetic Medication

You may hear alternative medicine advocates proclaim that the only thyroid drug anyone should take is *desiccated thyroid* such as Nature-Throid, WesThroid, or Armour Thyroid.

DEFINITION

Desiccated thyroid is prescription medication made from the cut-up and dried-out thyroid glands of pigs. It's the only medication available that contains all four thyroid hormones: T4 and T3 (in a 5:1 ratio), plus T2 and T1.

Other names for desiccated thyroid include *natural thyroid*, *glandular thyroid*, *natural desiccated thyroid*, and *NDT*.

However, most mainstream doctors automatically prescribe Synthroid, which is created from chemicals in a lab and contains only T4. If you request desiccated thyroid instead, many of these doctors will refuse, or at least give you a very hard time before saying yes.

This controversy results from a mix of historical and financial reasons. Synthroid first came on the market in 1955. Its manufacturer created an aggressive marketing campaign that touted it as new and modern, and portrayed desiccated thyroid as old-fashioned and inconsistent from batch to batch.

During this same period, there actually was a problem with a batch of desiccated thyroid that resulted in a patient being severely undertreated for hypothyroidism. This was reported in major medical journals, and it was the final straw that turned mainstream doctors away from natural thyroid to the new synthetic wonder. The problem was that the potency of desiccated thyroid medication at the time was determined by measuring iodine content. We now know this was a blunder, because the amount of iodine in a pill can vary independently of its active hormones—most notably, its T4 and T3 content. As a result, these medications truly *were* inconsistent.

Since the mid-1980s, though, desiccated thyroid manufacturers have switched to measuring the exact amounts of T4 and T3 in their pills. They follow the guidelines of the United States Pharmacopeia (USP), which is a highly respected authority that sets public standards for medication. Synthetic drug companies follow these same USP guidelines.

Therefore, while their ingredients come from different sources—pigs for natural thyroid and chemicals for synthetic—both types of pills are formulated in labs following strict quality control procedures, and you can expect to consistently get the stated amounts of T4 and/or T3 in a pill regardless of its origins.

However, Synthroid generates much more revenue. It costs up to four times as much as desiccated thyroid, and its manufacturer holds a patent on it, while pig thyroid isn't something anyone can patent. Some have observed that the greater financial clout of Synthroid's manufacturer has been used to influence medical organizations to tout it above all other thyroid solutions. In fact, Synthroid is one of the most-prescribed drugs in the United States.

Which isn't to say Synthroid isn't an excellent medication. It is. And for a large percentage of patients, the T4 it provides does the job. Their bodies convert the T4 into T3, and the latter supplies all the energy they need. Plus there are some clear advantages to Synthroid. Since it's made from lab-based ingredients that are never likely to run out, it's always readily available, while there have been periodic shortages of desiccated thyroid. Synthroid poses no problems for anyone who's uncomfortable consuming pig-based products, such as Orthodox Jews and vegetarians. And Synthroid is available in the widest range of dosages of all thyroid drugs, which makes it easy to fine-tune how much medication you're taking daily.

THYROID FACTOID

Synthroid is available in the following microgram (mcg) dosages and pill color codings to meet any need for T4: 25 mcg (orange), 50 mcg (white), 75 mcg (violet), 88 mcg (olive), 100 mcg (yellow), 112 mcg (rose), 125 mcg (brown), 137 mcg (turquoise), 150 mcg (blue), 175 mcg (lilac), 200 mcg (pink), and 300 mcg (green). And in case you can't remember what a color represents, the pertinent dosage number is etched into each pill.

However, a healthy thyroid produces not only T4, but also T3 (in a roughly 10:1 ratio). No one knows why, but it turns out that a large number of people really do need direct T3 as well as the T3 converted from T4. (This is especially the case for patients whose symptoms include depression, as direct T3 often has an enormous beneficial impact on emotions.) The solution for these patients is to take medication that provides direct T3 in addition to T4.

If you are one of these patients and your doctor won't budge from prescribing synthetics, you can request that your Synthroid be supplemented with Cytomel, which is synthetic T3. Cytomel's strength starts to fade after about 10 hours, so it should ideally be taken twice a day (once in the morning and once in the late afternoon). For many patients, a Synthroid-Cytomel mix is a great solution.

That said, a healthy thyroid also produces a certain amount of T2. There haven't been any major studies of T2 yet, but what's out there so far indicates that it plays a significant role in metabolism and weight loss. Studies also show that, all things being equal, patients taking synthetic medication have less than half the T2 of patients on desiccated thyroid. In other words, even if your body is converting T4 to T3 efficiently, it's probably not also converting enough of that T3 to T2. The only medication on the market that provides T2 is desiccated thyroid.

(Desiccated thyroid also contains T1, which doesn't appear to do anything useful, but it might serve some function no one's discovered yet.)

Therefore, if you're not feeling satisfied with the results of purely synthetic medication, you shouldn't hesitate to switch to desiccated thyroid—or, if you need to fine-tune your dosage, to a combination of Synthroid and desiccated thyroid. (There's no problem with mixing these medications; it's analogous to getting your daily vitamin C from eating two oranges, or by eating one orange and taking a vitamin pill.)

Alternatively, if you're seeing an open-minded doctor, you can simply start out with desiccated thyroid. It's much less expensive, just as reliable as Synthroid, and is the only medication that provides a mix of all four thyroid hormones.

There's no right or wrong answer to this controversy. People have different body chemistries, and also diverse relationships with their doctors. The way to find the best medication for you is to simply try out various options until all your symptoms disappear and you feel 100 percent well again.

Brand Name vs. Generic Medication

If you're using desiccated thyroid, you don't have to make brand name versus generic decisions. The brand names are already so inexpensive that no generics even exist.

If you're considering synthetic medication, though, such brands as Synthroid (T4) and Cytomel (T3) can be three times as expensive as their generic versions of levothyroxine (T4) and liothyronine (T3). Many patients swear they do significantly better on a particular brand name medication. Sometimes this is just their imagination. A perfect example are those who passionately declare WesThroid superior to Nature-Throid, or vice versa. The truth is that both medications come from the same manufacturer, RLC Labs, and are identical.

They didn't start out that way. WesThroid (on the market since 1934) originally had filler ingredients that caused some patients allergic reactions, so in the 1960s RLC came out with a hypoallergenic version named Nature-Throid. Eventually RLC decided to do away with WesThroid's allergic filler, and use the exact same active and inactive ingredients for both medications.

That doesn't mean patients who champion WesThroid over Nature-Throid are lying, though; the strength of their belief that one brand is superior to the other actually gives them a better experience with that brand.

Then again, sometimes patients really *are* better off with a particular brand.

The active ingredients in thyroid pills are minute—a fraction of the size of a grain of salt. Most of a thyroid pill therefore consists of inactive ingredients that serve as filler. While the active ingredients are the same in both brand name and generic versions, the fillers will vary … and will have different effects on how well or poorly the active ingredients are absorbed by your body.

Further, the same pill might be absorbed efficiently by you but badly by someone else, because each person's body chemistry is unique. (In fact, this is why you're told to take your thyroid medication 30-60 minutes before eating. Anything you consume might unexpectedly bond with the medication and prevent it from being absorbed.)

Therefore, the main advantage of buying a brand name is that you know what to expect. Unless the manufacturer changes the formulation, your pills will contain the same inactive ingredients every month; so even if you aren't absorbing a pill with maximum efficiency, it won't matter because your doctor will simply raise your dosage until you're always getting the amount of medication you need.

If you buy generic, though, there's a chance your pharmacy will obtain your pills from a different source in any given month. That means you could absorb the active ingredients efficiently one month and poorly the next—effectively changing your dosage without your knowledge.

That said, if you give generics a chance, you may find your body isn't very sensitive to changes to inactive ingredients. Or you may discover that your local pharmacy uses the same generic source month after month, in which case it'll provide you with the same consistency as the brand name version.

If you want to save $10-$30 a month, you're not at great risk by giving generics a try. But if you go this route, pay extra attention to how you're feeling; and don't hesitate to see your doctor for another blood test if you believe your symptoms might be returning.

THYROID FACTOID

There are occasional manufacturing snafus that cause a thyroid medication to be recalled, or to be temporarily taken off the market. This happens regardless of whether a thyroid medication is natural or synthetic, or a brand name or generic. The issue isn't the source of the hormones, but the extreme precision required to make *any* thyroid pill that meets or exceeds USP specifications.

Standard vs. Compounded Medication

Some doctors aren't satisfied with thyroid drugs as they come from their manufacturers, and instead have a local compounding pharmacy create a version customized to their specifications—typically, by putting the medication into a time-released form so it's more effective throughout the day. The reasoning is that while T4 is long-lasting, T3 loses its optimal strength relatively quickly.

However, if you're on desiccated thyroid medication such as Nature-Throid, the T3 will typically last most of the day; and since you're taking it daily, that's good enough.

Alternatively, if you're on Cytomel, its T3 will stop being optimal in your system after around 10 hours. If you find yourself fading out in the middle of the day, though, you can address this by taking half your Cytomel dosage in the morning and the other half in the late afternoon.

It's true that a compounded thyroid medication that's time-released provides extra convenience. But the risk isn't worth it. For example, a patient of mine we'll call

Stella was doing well on standard thyroid medication. She then became convinced by another doctor that he had better ideas and switched to him. A few months later I received a call from Stella over the weekend, and it quickly become obvious to me that she was suffering from severe hyperthyroid symptoms. I urged Stella to go straight to the ER. When she was admitted, the hospital found her T3 levels were hundreds of times above normal. Stella ended up spending several months in a coma and on a respirator, and for a while it didn't seem as if she'd survive.

What happened is that the other doctor prescribed Stella a compounded mixture of T3 in a time-released form. The dosage was supposed to be 7.5 micrograms. However, the pharmacist made a mistake and instead created a dosage of 7.5 *milligrams*, or *one thousand times* as much. You may wonder how such a blunder could happen, but both a milligram and a microgram are smaller than a grain of salt. When dealing with such minute quantities, errors can and do occur. In fact, Stella was lucky. Other patients have died from similar accidents with compounded thyroid medication.

It's possible you'll end up taking thyroid medication every day for the rest of your life. If so, using compounded medication means you'd be allowing 365 chances a year for a pharmacist to make a serious mistake. Considering that the convenience factor is small and there's a risk of a fatal outcome, I recommend staying away from compounded thyroid medication.

To be clear, there's nothing wrong with compounding pharmacies. Most other medications aren't in quantities as minute as thyroid hormones and so don't involve the same degree of danger. Also, not every doctor who prescribes compounded thyroid is a quack. Some just haven't thought through the ramifications. Still, if you're considering a doctor who follows this practice, take an extra careful look at what else that doctor is doing.

Thyroid Medication Substitutes

As you cruise the web or visit health food stores, you may find people touting over-the-counter substitutes for thyroid medication. These products are desiccated thyroid derived from pigs or cows, but with the fat extracted. Hormones are concentrated in the fatty acid of the glands, so removing the fat eliminates most of these products' active hormones. Obviously, that makes these products much less effective. If the bulk of the active hormones were allowed to remain, however, the USDA would consider these products drugs—which means you wouldn't be able buy them over the counter.

The ingredient lists of these substitutes imply that if you consumed about a dozen tablets, you'd be getting the rough equivalent of 1 grain (65 mg) of Nature-Throid. Even if that's true, it's a pretty inelegant way of taking thyroid medication. More importantly, these products aren't regulated remotely close to the standard of thyroid medication, so the dosing is likely to be inconsistent.

Also, because cow thyroid is sometimes used, and that thyroid is exposed to the brain during the slaughtering process, there's a small but real risk of contracting bovine spongiform encephalopathy (commonly known as mad cow disease). In other words, desiccated thyroid is a great product … but only via prescription.

Finally, as a general rule of thumb, it's not a good idea to self-medicate. You should work with a doctor who can regularly check your blood's thyroid levels and provide an objective view of your symptoms.

Other Over-the-Counter Remedies

There are also a number of over-the-counter products that claim to enhance thyroid function. The most popular are focused around iodine, which truly is a key component for thyroid hormone production. The only problem is these products often provide way *too much* iodine.

Specifically, you should consume between 150 and 300 mcg of iodine per day. You'll typically get at least 50-100 mcg automatically from the foods you eat, so you shouldn't even think about taking an iodine supplement that provides more than 200 mcg. However, many of these products provide doses of 1,000-50,000 mcg, which is utterly dangerous to your health.

If you want to supplement your iodine intake, some safe and tasty alternatives to consider are:

- **Nori:** Green seafood popular in Japan that's used to wrap sushi. It's also a fine snack.

- **Wakame:** Green seaweed with a subtly sweet flavor that's been farmed for centuries in Japan and Korea. You can use it in soups and salads.

- **Dulse:** Red algae that grows along the shorelines of the Atlantic and Pacific oceans, and tastes a little like beef jerky. It's an especially popular snack in Ireland and Iceland.

- **Iodized salt:** Table salt mixed with a tiny amount of iodine. You can sprinkle this on food as a quick and painless way to meet your iodine requirements.

Another safe way to add iodine is via a quality multivitamin pill, which will typically supply 50-100 mcg.

Also be aware that if you're taking Nature-Throid or WesThroid, 130 mcg of iodine is included in each 1 grain pill, which is as much supplemental iodine as you need.

The Least You Need to Know

- Steer clear of basal temperature testing, T3 overdoses, and iodine overdoses.
- To get all four thyroid hormones, take desiccated thyroid, either by itself or combined with synthetic thyroid.
- Avoid compounded thyroid medication.
- Don't buy poorly regulated over-the-counter thyroid remedies; stick to prescription thyroid medication.

Choosing the Right Doctor

In This Chapter

- Types of doctors to consider
- Identifying poor diagnostic attitudes
- Checking advice against lab results
- Identifying poor treatment approaches

Most major illnesses tend to be handled consistently and well throughout the medical community. In these cases you don't have to worry about which doctor to choose, because you're likely to receive a comparable level of care from any good doctor.

Unfortunately, that's not the situation when it comes to thyroid disorders, which can make even skilled and caring physicians fumble. Thyroid diagnosis and treatment is a moving target, and what doctors are taught in medical school doesn't always match up with the best practices of thyroid experts. Further, because the thyroid can cause any of dozens of seemingly unrelated symptoms, it's easy for doctors who aren't highly experienced with the thyroid to misinterpret the cause of a patient's problems ... or even dismiss those problems as being nothing more than the patient's imagination.

As a result, if you don't take an active role in ensuring you have the right thyroid practitioner for your needs, you may be playing Russian roulette with your health. This chapter guides you in understanding your options, what questions you should ask, and what behavior from your doctor indicates you're receiving optimal care.

Initial Considerations

If you have reason to suspect a thyroid disorder—for example, if you have several of the symptoms described in Chapter 2—you should get your blood checked to determine your thyroid's status. Specifically, your doctor should take a blood sample and send it to a lab, instructing the lab to test for at least three things: TSH, free T4, and free T3. The meaning of these tests are detailed in Chapter 7 (for hypothyroidism) and Chapter 11 (for hyperthyroidism). For now, what you need to know is that some less savvy doctors will order only a TSH test; but the TSH, free T4, and free T3 tests are *all* required to provide adequate information about your thyroid's condition.

In addition, a sharp doctor will usually tell the lab to perform a one-time check for thyroid antibodies. These are indicators of such conditions as Hashimoto's and Graves, which are the most frequent causes of thyroid disease.

Virtually any doctor can take your blood and send it to a lab, so you may find it easiest to begin with a general practitioner you already know and trust. Then again, if you want to be in the hands of a specialist from the start, you should seek out an *endocrinologist.*

DEFINITION

An **endocrinologist** is a doctor who specializes in disorders of the glands of the endocrine system and their hormones. These glands include the thyroid, parathyroids, pancreas, ovaries, testes, adrenal, pineal, pituitary, and hypothalamus.

For example, the most common illness treated by endocrinologists is diabetes, which is typically caused by the pancreas not producing enough insulin. And the next most common illness is hypothyroidism, which is typically caused by the thyroid not producing enough thyroid hormones.

Regardless of the type of doctor you see, your physician should carefully question you about your symptoms, conduct a thorough physical examination of your thyroid, and perform at least a brief overall physical exam.

If your doctor then wants to run tests beyond the thyroid blood tests, that's fine. In fact, it's often the responsible thing to do, because your symptoms might be stemming from something that has nothing do with your thyroid. Alternatively, they could be caused by multiple problems that include but aren't exclusive to your thyroid.

Here are some early warning signs that should make you seriously consider switching to a different doctor:

- You're told to ignore a symptom—"It's just in your head" or "Reduce your stress and it'll go away." It's possible that's true, but there's no way to be sure until you're tested.

- You're told the only tests you need don't involve your thyroid. It's fine to test for other things, but *in addition* to checking your thyroid hormone levels. Thyroid tests are only around $50 each, and are covered by virtually all insurance plans, so there's no good reason to not perform them.

- You're told that the only thyroid test needed is the TSH test. That's the sign of a doctor out of touch with modern thyroid diagnosis methods. You can either insist on having free T4, free T3, and thyroid antibody tests included until the doctor complies, or you can say "thanks but no thanks" and seek a physician with more up-to-date knowledge.

If your doctor doesn't do any of these things, then you're probably in good hands. Before you end your visit, however, ask if you can be faxed the thyroid test results after they come in from the lab. Be tactful when making this request, indicating that you know a little about what the numbers mean (which you will after reading Chapter 7 or Chapter 11), and you're simply eager to get some idea of your thyroid's condition ASAP.

If your practitioner seems a bit put off by the request, that's not unusual, as doctors are accustomed to being fully in charge. But dealing with thyroid issues is a genuine collaboration between doctor and patient, and the best thyroid practitioners understand that. Be polite and diplomatic, and there shouldn't be a problem.

If your doctor flat-out refuses, that's another warning sign. In this case, ask if you can alternatively receive a photocopy of the results when you come in for your next visit. If you receive another no, then cancel the test and seek another doctor. You own your medical information and are legally entitled to it upon request. A doctor who denies your right to your lab data is also likely to deny your right to participate in your treatment.

THYROIDIAN TIP

If you don't have a fax machine, you can get faxes e-mailed to you as PDF attachments. Some services will do this for free for the first 30 days and/or as long as you don't exceed a 20-page limit (which is no problem, as your test results will typically fit on 1-3 pages). Alternatively, if you need ongoing fax capabilities, an especially good and inexpensive service is MyFax.com. To learn more, Google the phrase *Best fax services.*

Note: If your doctor detects one or more noticeable growths on your thyroid—that is, large enough to be seen and/or felt in your neck—then regardless of the results of the blood test, you must have these checked out, too. Your doctor can begin by prescribing an ultrasound exam, which is quick, inexpensive, and poses no health risks. If the results don't clearly show the growths to be benign, there's a small possibility of thyroid cancer. For safety's sake, you should therefore follow up by seeing an experienced ear, nose, and throat surgeon (see Chapter 13).

Your Second Visit

If you asked for your thyroid test results to be faxed to you, then typically within a few days you'll receive a page with some numbers on it from your doctor's office.

To understand these results, read Chapter 7 (if you think you're hypothyroid) or Chapter 11 (if you suspect hyperthyroidism). It will explain:

- What all the test numbers mean.
- The TSH range used by the lab, which we'll call the *broad range.*
- The TSH range that savvy thyroid experts use, which we'll call the *narrow range.*

If your TSH falls within the narrow range, then you probably don't have a thyroid problem. If your TSH falls outside of the broad range, then you probably do; and your doctor won't need any convincing to treat you with thyroid medication.

If your TSH falls between the narrow and broad range, however, you're in a gray area that will make your diagnosis complicated. In this case your doctor should pay extra careful attention to your free T3 and free T4 results; and more importantly, she should look beyond the numbers to your symptoms. If your symptoms persist, and no other clear cause is identified for them, then you should be treated for thyroid disease regardless of the lab numbers. There's no significant downside to treatment; and if you really do have a thyroid problem, then within 2-6 weeks you should start feeling better.

Having this knowledge makes you an informed patient, and empowers you to both understand and evaluate your doctor's choices. When you see your doctor again, listen carefully as she discusses your thyroid test results, and notice whether what she's telling you matches up with your own understanding. If you're confused, don't be shy about asking questions. (Sometimes doctors make shocking mistakes—for example, interpreting a high TSH to mean you have high thyroid levels, when it actually means the opposite.)

If your TSH happens to fall into the gray area between the narrow and broad ranges, also pay attention to whether your doctor dismisses the possibility that you have thyroid disease. If this occurs, mention that the TSH range recommended by the American Association of Clinical Endocrinologists (AACE) indicates you're at risk, and that you don't believe your symptoms are just your imagination. If your doctor dismisses this as well, then you need to find another doctor.

Alternatively, if your physician demonstrates she has a balanced view by taking both the lab numbers and your symptoms into consideration, and by not treating the lab's recommended ranges as gospel, then the chances are she's the right doctor for you.

Considering Treatment Options

If your doctor decides that you need thyroid treatment, then your next discussion should be about medication. If you're seeing a mainstream doctor, he'll probably prescribe Synthroid (or the generic version levothyroxine), which is lab-created T4. Most patients will do fine on Synthroid. However, many others—in my experience, as many as one out of three—will not.

The problem is that a healthy thyroid produces both T4 and T3 (in a 10:1 ratio), but Synthroid is exclusively T4. Many patients will therefore do better on a mix of Synthroid and Cytomel (which is lab-created T3), or on desiccated thyroid such as Nature-Throid (which is natural thyroid taken from pigs, providing a mix of T4, T3, T2, and T1). More information about these medications can be found in Chapters 3 and 8.

Therefore, it's not inappropriate to ask your doctor to add Cytomel to the Synthroid; or to skip the synthetic route altogether and start off with desiccated thyroid. If he scoffs at the request and replies that Synthroid will always be the best choice, then he's not giving you accurate advice, but don't be too hard on him; he's merely echoing what he was taught in medical school. If you find he's a good doctor in all other ways, then you may want to give him a chance and see if you do well on the Synthroid.

One exception is if your thyroid has entirely stopped functioning or has been removed, in which case you're relying exclusively on your medication to provide the thyroid hormones your body requires. In this case you're really better off with desiccated thyroid medication such as Nature-Throid, because it's the only option that will provide you with the full range of thyroid hormones—that is, T4, T3, T2, and T1. If your doctor won't agree to your preference for medication, then you can start on Synthroid (which will do no harm), but also begin looking around for a different practitioner who'll accommodate you.

If you need help locating an appropriate doctor in your area, use the website resources listed in Appendix B. These range from online patient recommendations of thyroid doctors to free searchable databases containing information on hundreds of thousands of physicians.

THYROIDIAN TIP

If your mainstream doctor won't prescribe desiccated thyroid, you can find alternative doctors who will through the American Association of Naturopathic Physicians. Its website at Naturopathic.org allows you to search for doctors by specialty (select *Adrenal Fatigue/Endocrinology*) or by state. You can also get recommendations for alternative doctors through compounding pharmacies in your area, as these pharmacies typically stock desiccated thyroid. This is a bit tricky, however, because you don't want a doctor who prescribes compounded thyroid medication (see Chapter 3).

Follow-Up Visits

Once you've begun treatment, your doctor should see you every 1-2 months until your condition appears to be stable.

First, your doctor should keep taking your blood to check your TSH, free T4, and free T3 levels. The initial dosage you were given was simply your doctor's best guess. These subsequent visits will allow your doctor to fine-tune your dosage based on your test results. This is a trial-and-error process, so it may take months of mild adjustments until your doctor finds the prescription that's perfect for you. Detailed information about dosages appears in Chapter 9.

In addition, at each visit your doctor should perform a quick physical exam and question you about how you're feeling. If your symptoms are getting increasingly less severe, or have entirely disappeared, then the medication is working. But if that's not happening, you shouldn't hesitate to say so. What really matters aren't lab numbers but whether your symptoms are being successfully treated. The latter is the most important indicator of your health and what your doctor should focus on.

If your doctor refuses to make treatment adjustments even though your symptoms show no signs of improvement, then have a frank discussion about your concerns. If you aren't satisfied by your doctor's answers, seek a more diligent practitioner.

Beware Extremists

A thyroid doctor who takes a hard-line approach in any direction is likely to be problematic. This chapter has already warned against mainstream doctors who believe Synthroid is the only appropriate medication for all thyroid patients. But you should also be wary of alternative doctors who proclaim that Nature-Throid is the only acceptable treatment. For example, if you require a finely tuned combination of T4 and T3, then a mix of Synthroid and Nature-Throid, or Synthroid and Cytomel, may prove to be ideal.

Here are some other approaches from alternative thyroid doctors that should set off alarm bells:

- **No blood tests.** If a doctor claims blood tests are unreliable, he's living in the 1950s. Thyroid tests really were lacking decades ago, but modern tests are accurate and invaluable tools.

- **Prescribing iodine overdoses.** There's no solid evidence that excessive iodine does any good; and there's reason to believe it's dangerous, raising the risk of developing Graves' disease, Hashimoto's disease, or thyroid cancer.

- **Prescribing way too little thyroid medication.** Some doctors outrageously underprescribe; for example, by telling patients to take their thyroid medication once a week instead of daily. This not only fails to cure symptoms, but stresses the endocrine system more than if no medication was provided.

- **Prescribing way too much thyroid medication.** You typically shouldn't take much more than 1 mcg of T4 per pound of your body weight. Some alternative doctors instruct their patients to take four, five, or even six times as much thyroid medication as necessary. Over time this puts patients into a hyperthyroid state, which can lead to heart failure, accelerated osteoporosis, and other deadly disorders.

- **Treating reverse T3.** Some alternative doctors subscribe to a theory called Wilson's syndrome that focuses on a byproduct of T4 called reverse T3, and they treat it with T3 megadoses. There's no solid evidence to support these ideas, and the treatment is so dangerous that it's caused deaths. Stay away.

- **Prescribing compounded medication.** There's usually nothing wrong with compounded drugs—that is, medication prepared by a local pharmacy to a doctor's specifications. It's dangerous when it comes to thyroid medication, however, because the active ingredients in thyroid pills are so minute that even a small mistake by a pharmacist can result in an enormous overdose. Patients have died from such errors.

Additional details about these practices appear in Chapter 3. The bottom line is you should steer clear of doctors with these wrong-headed approaches, which have little connection to medical science and can put your health at serious risk.

THROAT QUOTE

In the history of mankind, fanaticism has caused more harm than vice.

—Louis Kronenberger

Instead, look for a doctor who has is open-minded and has a balanced approach. If you're exploring mainstream doctors, look for one who isn't focused solely on lab results, but also pays careful attention to your symptoms and to how you're feeling. And if you're considering alternative doctors, look for one who makes full use of modern medical tools such as thyroid blood tests and doesn't advocate wacky theories.

When it comes to thyroid care, a nuanced, middle-ground approach produces the best results.

The Least You Need to Know

- Ask your doctor to test your TSH, free T3, free T4, and thyroid antibody levels.
- Ask for your test results to be faxed to you so you can study them before your next doctor's visit.
- Seek a doctor who'll pay attention to your symptoms as well as your lab results.
- Follow up for trial-and-error testing to achieve your optimal dosage.

Hypothyroidism

In this part we focus on hypothyroidism, which is typically caused by an underactive thyroid, and comprises the vast majority of thyroid disease cases. We explore potential causes for the disease, describe its symptoms, and discuss other diseases that have similar symptoms in case you have one of them instead of—or in addition to—a thyroid problem.

Chapter 7 explains the key thyroid blood tests you need, and details how to obtain and analyze your lab results. Chapter 8 tells you about your medication options, and why what most doctors automatically prescribe may not be the best choice. And Chapter 9 guides you through the process of determining your perfect dosage for optimal health.

Types of Hypothyroidism

In This Chapter

- Causes and effects of Hashimoto's disease
- How goiters grow
- Becoming hypothyroid despite a healthy thyroid
- How doctors and drugs can make you hypothyroid
- The dangers of iodine overdosing

If you're gaining weight, feeling fatigued, losing hair, becoming depressed, or experiencing any of dozens of other symptoms, you may be *hypothyroid*. Hypothyroidism accounts for four out of five cases of thyroid disease. Over 24 million Americans are estimated to have hypothyroidism, and hundreds of millions of people suffer from it worldwide.

What Is Hypothyroidism?

As explained in Chapter 1, your thyroid regulates the energy level of every cell in your body through the production of its hormones. Hypothyroidism occurs when the levels of those hormones—primarily T3 and T4—are below normal. In fact, the first part of this disease's name, *hypo*, is Greek for *below* (just as *hypo*dermic refers to injections below the skin).

The lack of hormones reduces the activity and regeneration of cells throughout your body. This lowered metabolism can result in dramatic weight gain, sluggishness, confusion, insomnia, lowered sex drive, dry nails and skin, feeling cold, and/or myriad other problems. (For a more complete list, see Chapter 6.)

Hypothyroidism can range from mild thyroid underperformance—resulting in symptoms so subtle you don't consciously notice them—to a total shutdown of your thyroid. You can even be hypothyroid if your thyroid is healthy. For example, a defective pituitary gland can order your thyroid to underperform (as we'll explain shortly), or T3 can be blocked from "powering up" your cells by ailing adrenal glands (see Chapter 14).

Hypothyroidism is a complicated disease. On the one hand, it's easy to treat because inexpensive prescription medication will very effectively replace whatever thyroid hormones you lack. On the other hand, hypothyroidism is often difficult to recognize because its group of wildly diverse symptoms can seem to have nothing to do with each other. Even experienced doctors who don't happen to be thyroid experts often fail to properly diagnose it. The American Association of Clinical Endocrinologists (AACE) estimates that half of those with hypothyroidism don't know it—making this widespread disease a quiet epidemic.

Adding to the problem is the fact most doctors are taught in medical school to prescribe T4-only medication across the board. However, many patients require a mix of T4 and T3 to fully resolve their symptoms. Further, even if you're taking the right medication, it can be tricky to arrive at the precise dosage for achieving optimum health.

This is the first of five chapters providing you with the knowledge you need to meet the various challenges posed by hypothyroidism. Once you've read these chapters, you'll know whether you should see a doctor; and how to make sure you receive the best testing, diagnosis, and treatment.

Hashimoto's Disease

In underdeveloped countries, the primary cause of hypothyroidism is insufficient iodine. In countries such as the United States where iodine is plentiful, however, roughly 75-85 percent of hypothyroidism results from *Hashimoto's disease*. This exotic-sounding illness is named after Hashimoto Hakaru, a Japanese doctor who in 1912 was the first to publish a medical analysis of it. Hashimoto's strikes women over five times as often as men; and the odds of getting it increase as you grow older.

Causes of Hashimoto's Disease

Hashimoto's is an autoimmune disease. It occurs when your immune system—which normally protects you by attacking foreign invaders such as bacteria and viruses—mistakes your thyroid as a danger and starts attacking it, too.

Hashimoto's is typically caused by a genetic disposition for an autoimmune problem coupled with a trigger that pushes the immune system over the edge. No one is certain what the primary trigger for Hashimoto's is, but the current best guess of experts is a buildup of toxic environmental chemicals in the thyroid.

Your thyroid is especially sensitive to chemicals because it's designed to sift through your blood, and suck in and store even the tiniest amounts of iodine it finds. This ability of your thyroid is normally wonderful, because it means you need to consume only a little bit of iodine for your thyroid to have enough of it to make its hormones.

The problem is that over the last 100 years our world has become flooded with chemicals. According to the U.S. Environmental Protection Agency there are more than 100,000 chemicals in commercial use, and over 2,300 new ones submitted to the EPA for approval every year.

Some of these substances are designed to be toxic—for example, the pesticides used to keep insects away from crops. Others include cheap and mildly toxic substances in products that aren't eaten, but nonetheless get through your skin and into your bloodstream (this happens a lot with cosmetics). Yet others become toxic as a processing side effect, such as the corn syrup that some factories make using mercury-based components, which recent testing has found results in small amounts of mercury turning up in thousands of snacks and beverages.

> **THROAT QUOTE**
>
> Give a man a fish, and he can eat for a day. But teach a man how to fish, and he'll be dead of mercury poisoning inside of three years.
>
> —Charles Haas

The amount of any commercial chemical you're exposed to is supposed to be small enough to be safe. But many of these substances haven't been around long enough for us to know what their long-term effects will be. Just as importantly, no one knows how you'll be affected by the combination of hundreds of chemicals in your daily life that have never been tested together.

This is relevant to your thyroid because the same mechanism that allows it to draw in and store tiny amounts of iodine from your bloodstream also leads it to extract and store toxins you consume that happen to be chemically similar to iodine. The latter include mercury (which is poisonous) and perchlorate (which is used in such products as rocket fuel, and is often present in low-quality drinking water).

The iodine in your thyroid eventually gets used up in the production of hormones, but the toxins don't. So even though your thyroid is taking in very small quantities of toxins, they'll accumulate decade after decade. This means the longer you live, the more likely the toxins you're exposed to will accumulate to serious levels (which is why the risk of developing Hashimoto's increases with age). At some point the amount of toxins in your thyroid can become so significant that they'll trigger your body's immune system. Your antibodies (specifically, *thyroid peroxidase* and/or *thyroglobulin* antibodies) will designate them as unwelcome invaders, and multiply to assault the cells containing them and flush them out of your system.

Unfortunately, what often happens is the antibodies will mistake your healthy thyroid cells as being a threat along with the cells harboring toxins. The antibodies will respond by attacking your whole thyroid; there's no practical way to stop them. (Your doctor could shut down your immune system, but that would be a "cure" worse than the threat to your thyroid.)

However, if you're in the early stages of Hashimoto's, you might be able to mitigate the situation—or at least avoid making it worse—by cutting toxins out of your life as much as possible. For details, see Chapters 18 and 22.

While environmental toxins paired with a genetic disposition are believed to be the primary cause of Hashimoto's, there are a couple of other significant ways the disease can be triggered. The most abrupt one is a respiratory infection that induces your body to create numerous antibodies to combat it. Sometimes antibodies looking for invaders in your neck will become confused and end up attacking your thyroid—which will begin the chain of events leading to Hashimoto's. You can also develop Hashimoto's as a result of iodine overdoses, which at high enough levels can be perceived as toxic by your immune system.

Effects of Hashimoto's Disease

The effects of chronic Hashimoto's assaults vary for different people. If you have a mild case, the disease may reduce your thyroid's ability to produce hormones by around 5 percent a year. In this situation the symptoms are so subtle and gradual that you may not realize you're sick for a long time. But once you begin taking thyroid medication, the numerous specific improvements you'll experience will make you suddenly aware of all the ways your body had gone wrong.

On the other hand, Hashimoto's might attack your thyroid aggressively. This could lead to your developing symptoms in an abrupt and very noticeable way. It could also lead to one or more *goiters*, which are enlargements of your thyroid.

In addition, Hashimoto's can cause temporary *hyper*thyroidism. While the disease will make you hypothyroid over the long term, in its early stages it kills a lot of healthy thyroid cells, and as these cells die, they'll spill out whatever hormones they contained. This can inject surges of T4 and T3 into your bloodstream, and bring about such symptoms of hyperthyroidism as a rapidly beating heart, anxiety, and panic attacks. You can obtain relief from these symptoms by taking medication for hyperthyroidism until this stage of the disease—which is called *Hashitoxicosis*—eventually ends and your Hashimoto's stabilizes into keeping you exclusively hypothyroid.

THYROIDIAN TIP

If Hashimoto's is giving you the worst of both worlds by alternately making you hypothyroid and hyperthyroid, your TSH levels may appear *normal* on blood tests. That's because the underproduction of thyroid hormones will be evened out by the hormone surges caused by slaughtered thyroid cells. It's therefore important that the initial lab testing your doctor orders for you includes antibody tests, which will pick up the presence of Hashimoto's regardless of your TSH levels.

Goitrous Hypothyroidism

A *goiter* is a non-cancerous swelling on your thyroid. Your thyroid can grow one goiter or multiple goiters. This condition isn't really a disease unto itself, but a side effect of other hypothyroid diseases such as Hashimoto's. Goiters happen when your body's low levels of thyroid hormones cause your pituitary gland to send out increasing amounts of TSH. Because your thyroid isn't capable of producing enough hormones to meet the pituitary's demands at its current size, it responds by growing more cells. This is an effective strategy under normal circumstances, but when disease or shortages are at play, it's doomed to failure.

For example, if you're suffering from an autoimmune disease such as Hashimoto's, the hostile chemical environment created by antibodies will prevent new thyroid cells from being capable of producing hormones. And for those suffering from insufficient iodine—which is the most common cause of goiters in underdeveloped countries—new cells won't help because the thyroid will still lack the iodine needed to construct T4 and T3 molecules. In such cases, your body will continue to lack thyroid hormones; your pituitary gland will keep yelling at your thyroid to do something about it; and your thyroid will hopelessly keep making its goiters bigger.

If your hypothyroidism is treated in its early stages, any goiters that may have developed will never become large enough to be felt or noticed. Once you go on thyroid medication and your hormone levels return to normal, your pituitary gland will stop overstimulating your thyroid and its goiters will simply stop growing.

If you've been hypothyroid for a long time without treatment, though, then one or more goiters may become large enough to become visible in your neck, and/or to cause you trouble when speaking, breathing, or swallowing. In fact, the primary value of goiters is to make themselves known in this way, because they provide undeniable evidence that your body has a chronic shortage of thyroid hormones that needs to be addressed.

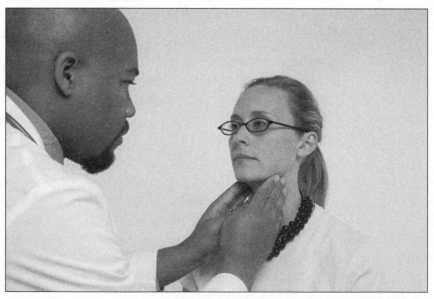

Checking the thyroid for goiters.
(Licensed from Shutterstock Images)

Once you're on thyroid medication, your goiters will probably go away over time. Your pituitary gland will not only stop stimulating their growth, but will stop encouraging the replacement of dying goiter cells with fresh ones, resulting in natural shrinkage. If your goiters don't disappear on their own, though, and if they're large enough to be uncomfortable and/or cosmetically displeasing, you can opt to have them surgically removed.

THYROIDIAN TIP

It's a good idea to check your neck periodically for growths, which could end up being harmless goiters or—much more rarely—cancer nodules (see Chapter 13). To do so, first get a handheld mirror and a glass of water. Then hold the mirror in front of you and, while keeping your eyes focused on the lower portion of your neck, drink the water. If you see any bulges that probably shouldn't be there when you swallow, visit your doctor to have them checked out. However, don't get confused by your Adam's apple; your thyroid is below it, closer to your collarbone.

Pituitary Gland Disease

As explained in Chapter 1, your pituitary gland manages the activity of your thyroid by producing TSH whenever your body needs additional thyroid hormones. Most cases of hypothyroidism result from an ailing thyroid being unable to entirely fulfill the orders represented by the TSH.

However, you can also become hypothyroid if your pituitary gland becomes ill and starts underproducing TSH. In this case, even though your thyroid is entirely healthy, it'll end up making too little T4 and T3 because that's effectively what it's being told to do.

This situation, called *pituitary disease*, can be picked up by standard thyroid blood tests. That's because when you're hypothyroid you'll normally have low thyroid hormone levels and high TSH levels—the latter being a result of your pituitary gland screaming, "Make more hormones!" If the problem is with your pituitary gland, though, you'll have low hormone levels *and* low TSH.

As a double check, your doctor can test the levels of other hormones regulated by your pituitary gland, such as those produced by your adrenal glands and sex glands. The chances are great that they'll be low as well.

The most common cause for your pituitary malfunctioning is developing a non-cancerous growth called an *adenoma*. If the adenoma is tiny—14 millimeters or less—your doctor will treat it with medication such as *Bromocriptine* that can slow, and even reverse, adenoma growth. If the adenoma is larger, though, then its continued growth risks putting dangerous pressure on your nearby optic nerves. In this situation, you should consider surgery to cut out the adenoma.

Therapeutic Hypothyroidism

No matter what type of thyroid disease you start out with, the chances are your doctors will cause you to end up hypothyroid. This is called *therapeutic hypothyroidism* because it results from treatment you receive for a thyroid disorder.

For example, if you're hyperthyroid, your treatment may involve surgery or radiation to reduce the size of your thyroid. In a perfect world, the reduction would be so precise that you'd end up with normal hormone production. In reality, though, your doctor will err on the side of making you mildly hypothyroid. That's because you're much safer being hypothyroid than hyperthyroid, and the hypothyroidism can be easily managed with medication.

As another—and more extreme—example, if you have thyroid cancer, you and your doctor may decide to surgically remove your entire thyroid. This will make you hypothyroid because your body will no longer have the ability to produce any thyroid hormones on its own. Once you start taking thyroid medication, however, your T4 and T3 levels will return to normal.

By far the most common scenario for therapeutic hypothyroidism is being on thyroid medication but remaining somewhat hypothyroid. This can happen if you're exclusively on a T4 prescription when your body happens to also require direct T3. It can also occur if you're taking the right medications but at dosages that are too low. In such cases, trust what you're feeling and observing. If your physician won't acknowledge that you're still hypothyroid, seek a doctor who'll focus on your symptoms instead of just your lab tests (see Chapter 4).

Drug-Induced Hypothyroidism

While therapeutic hypothyroidism stems from thyroid treatment, *drug-induced hypothyroidism* occurs when you become hypothyroid from medication that has nothing to do with your thyroid.

For example, patients taking lithium—typically for bipolar disorder—have a 50 percent chance of becoming hypothyroid and growing goiters as a side effect of the drug. That's because lithium is chemically similar enough to iodine that the thyroid may eventually start pulling it from the bloodstream and storing it—which then doesn't leave enough room for the thyroid to store adequate amounts of iodine. It's largely for this reason that lithium is no longer a doctor's first choice. However, it's still prescribed when other medications don't work.

An even more problematic drug is *amiodarone*, which is used to stabilize an irregular heartbeat. Amiodarone has a number of severe side effects, with hypothyroidism being among the milder ones.

> **THROAT QUOTE**
>
> I find the medicine worse than the malady.
>
> —John Fletcher

As a general rule, whenever your doctor prescribes a medication with which you aren't familiar, make a point of looking up its side effects, and then pay close attention to your body to see if any of them occur. This can be tricky with hypothyroidism since its symptoms aren't always obvious; so whenever you're in doubt, err on the side of caution and get your blood tested. If it turns out the drug is lowering your hormone levels, switch to another drug if possible, or start taking thyroid medication to make up for its effects.

Toxin-Induced Hypothyroidism

As explained previously, if your thyroid accumulates small amounts of toxins over a long time, it may develop Hashimoto's disease. However, it's also possible to take in a relatively large amount of toxins in a short period of time. If the toxins are chemically similar to iodine, then you'll become hypothyroid. In addition, you may experience severe symptoms beyond hypothyroidism. If the problem is detected early enough, though, treatment may spare you from any permanent damage.

For example, a patient named Dorothy came to me with pain in her muscles. Dorothy was used to starting a new exercise regime and having several days of muscle pain afterward. That's normal, but Dorothy was now experiencing this kind of pain in almost all her muscles, and all the time, even without exercising. Accompanying this were severe fatigue, trouble sleeping, and depression. When she came to me she was on antidepressants and pain medications, but her quality of life was pretty miserable.

I found Dorothy tested positive for hypothyroidism, and in addition had high levels of mercury in her blood. She underwent treatment to remove the mercury from her body, and also begin taking low doses of thyroid medication. Over time Dorothy felt enormously better, and was able to wean herself off all the antidepressant and pain medications. And because the problem was caused by toxins rather than a permanently defective thyroid, Dorothy was eventually able to wean herself off her thyroid medication as well.

Iodine-Induced Hypothyroidism

Some people have the notion that if a reasonable amount of a substance is good for you, then taking a lot of it will be even better. The opposite is usually true, and a prime example is iodine.

Your thyroid is dependent on iodine to make its hormones, but it needs only a small amount—150 to 300 micrograms a day. Staying in that range is safest; and you should definitely take no more than 1,000 mcg on any given day. But as explained in Chapter 3, there are both alternative medicine practitioners and over-the-counter products recommending daily iodine megadoses of 1,000-50,000 mcg. Not only is this not good for you, it'll probably make you hypothyroid.

The reason is a flood of iodine risks your thyroid abruptly making way too much of its hormones, a condition called a *thyroid storm*. This in turn puts you in jeopardy of going into such a severe hyperthyroid state that your heart pounds in your chest until you have a heart attack.

Your body understands this danger, so it "blows a fuse" when you feed it too much iodine by entirely shutting down your thyroid. Your thyroid won't start working again until your body flushes the excess iodine from your system over 2-3 weeks. If you pump extreme doses of iodine into your body day after day, though, you may keep your thyroid shut down long enough to do permanent damage to it.

Alternatively, your antibodies may perceive the excess iodine as a toxic invader, and start attacking both it and your thyroid cells. This can lead to Hashimoto's disease; or even worse, Graves' disease (see Chapter 10).

Excess iodine can also lead to growths on your thyroid. Sometimes these will be harmless goiters, but sometimes they end up being cancerous.

The way to avoid all this is simple: stay within the recommended range of 150-300 mcg of iodine a day. That means saying no to megadose iodine pills. And it also means being aware of the iodine content of what you consume. For example, a reasonable amount of seafood is terrific for you. Inexpensive and low-calorie natural iodine sources include fish, shellfish, and the seaweeds nori, wakame, and dulse. But if you eat a great deal of seafood daily, you may be taking in too much iodine. (In fact, seaside villages tend to have high rates of thyroid disease.)

As another example, if you're on the desiccated thyroid medications Nature-Throid or WesThroid, you're taking in 130 mcg of iodine with each 1 grain pill, which is all the supplemental iodine your body requires.

If you've been overdosing on iodine without realizing it, don't panic. The human body is resilient; and as long as you cut back to normal levels, you may well avoid any lasting damage.

The Least You Need to Know

- Hypothyroidism is a quiet epidemic, affecting over 24 million people in the United States and hundreds of millions worldwide.
- Hashimoto's disease can be triggered by genetics, environmental toxins, a respiratory infection, or iodine overdosing.
- Goiters are noncancerous growths on your thyroid resulting from a lack of thyroid hormones.
- Even if your thyroid is healthy, you can become hypothyroid from an underactive pituitary gland, insufficient iodine, or drugs chemically similar to iodine.
- Regardless of what type of thyroid disease initially strikes you, you'll probably end up hypothyroid.

Hypothyroidism Symptoms

6

In This Chapter

- Understanding hypothyroidism symptoms
- Checking off your symptoms
- True tales of hypothyroid patients
- Conditions with similar or parallel symptoms

Hypothyroidism is often hard to identify because it can create any of dozens of seemingly unrelated symptoms, ranging from abrupt weight gain to fatigue to hair loss to depression. Even excellent physicians who don't happen to be thyroid experts might not recognize when you're hypothyroid.

While Chapter 2 covered all thyroid diseases, this chapter focuses squarely on hypothyroidism. It begins with a checklist of symptoms to help you decide if you're hypothyroid. It then provides some real-life stories about patients who thoroughly overcame hypothyroid problems with inexpensive medication.

In addition, it briefly describes other common conditions that resemble and/or overlap with hypothyroidism, which will help you both clarify what your symptoms are and decide what tests to request when you see your doctor.

Once you're done reading, you'll have a checklist of symptoms you can take to your doctor for testing, diagnosis, and possible treatment.

I was so exhausted I couldn't figure out what was going on in my life. I ended up going to Africa and spent a month with my beautiful daughters there, was still feeling really tired, really tired, going around from doctor to doctor trying to figure out what was wrong.

—Oprah Winfrey on her hypothyroidism

Acknowledging Symptoms

Your thyroid regulates your energy levels by producing hormones that allow your cells to stay "powered up" and active, and to grow and generate new cells. Since every part of your body requires energy, if your thyroid starts underproducing these hormones you may experience any number of issues involving your skin, your hair, your brain, your sexual organs, and more.

Some symptoms may be obvious, such as sudden weight gain or severe tiredness. Others may be so subtle—such as feeling confused or less interested in sex—that you're unlikely to immediately recognize them as the results of an illness.

Diagnosing hypothyroidism is tricky for doctors as well. Different patients can have completely different symptoms, combinations of symptoms, and severities of symptoms, all stemming from an off-kilter thyroid. While most hypothyroid issues aren't immediately serious, they can become dangerous over time. And either way, they have a significant negative impact on quality of life.

There are millions of people who suffer with debilitating problems simply because neither they nor their doctors have recognized the root cause as insufficient thyroid hormones. It's a tragedy, because you can easily make up for any lack of T4 and T3 with inexpensive pills … but not until your hypothyroidism has been identified.

Too often we rationalize changes in our bodies, altering our perception of what's normal instead of acknowledging there's something wrong. This chapter will empower you to listen to your body when it's saying your thyroid is underperforming.

Hypothyroidism Symptoms Checklist

Because thyroid hormones affect every cell, in theory an underactive thyroid can result in any of hundreds of symptoms. In general, though, certain symptoms are more likely to occur than others. These frequent clues to hypothyroidism appear in the checklist that follows.

Take a few minutes to go over the list and check off any symptom that applies to you. If you aren't sure whether you have a particular symptom, find the description of it in Chapter 2 and use the additional information to make your decision.

Hypothyroidism Symptoms Checklist

- ❏ Gaining weight for no apparent reason
- ❏ Frequent exhaustion
- ❏ Sluggishness
- ❏ Slowed thinking
- ❏ Memory problems
- ❏ Depression
- ❏ Lowered interest in sex
- ❏ Menstrual problems
- ❏ Infertility
- ❏ Insomnia
- ❏ Constipation
- ❏ Hair loss
- ❏ Thinning or dry hair
- ❏ Dry, brittle nails
- ❏ Rough, itchy, and/or thinning skin
- ❏ Acne
- ❏ Puffy skin
- ❏ Cold skin
- ❏ Feeling unusually cold
- ❏ Sweating too little
- ❏ Numbness in the hands and feet
- ❏ Weak muscles
- ❏ Hoarse voice
- ❏ Enlarged neck

If you have six or more of these common symptoms, there's a strong chance you're hypothyroid. Get your thyroid checked out—typically via blood tests for TSH, free T4, free T3, and antibodies—as soon as possible.

If you have two to five of these symptoms, that's still reason enough to get your thyroid tested. Either the results will be positive, putting you on the path to treatment, or negative, which will inform your doctor to explore other potential problem sources. (Before accepting a negative result, though, see Chapter 7.) But even if you have only one of these symptoms and your doctor isn't providing a satisfying explanation for its cause, you should seriously consider getting tested. That's especially true if you're a woman 30 to 50 years old, as that's the gender and age range most often struck by hypothyroidism.

The checklist is by no means comprehensive; you can definitely experience other symptoms. However, the odds are that along with the unlisted symptoms you'll have at least a few of the ones on the checklist.

If you're successfully treated, you'll soon experience improvement regarding *all* your hypothyroidism symptoms.

THROAT QUOTE

I was depressed, I kept gaining weight, and I had no interest in sex. My doctor sent me to a psychiatrist, but that didn't help at all. Then my hair started falling out.

—Patient who fully recovered after going on thyroid medication

Hypothyroid Patient Stories

It can be easier to understand symptoms when they're viewed within the context of people's lives. The following are true stories of people struggling with medical problems that turned out to be the results of hypothyroidism. Most of these patients had been misdiagnosed before they turned to me for help. They were all restored to full health via inexpensive thyroid medication.

Memory Problems

JoAnne was a delightful woman in her early 70s who abruptly began suffering from impaired mental functioning. JoAnne used to enjoy moderating Civil War discussion groups and traveling to historic battlegrounds, but her memory suddenly became so poor that she gave up all such activities. JoAnne's children were concerned she was experiencing dementia or early Alzheimer's, and had made an appointment for her to see a neurologist. She came to me first in hopes of discovering a more treatable cause.

When I started asking JoAnne questions, it became clear that she wasn't only losing her memory but her enthusiasm for life. She told me her best friend had switched from calling her a spitfire to calling her an old dishrag. Thyroid testing was definitely called for.

JoAnne proved to be very clearly hypothyroid. Medication quickly turned things around. It's fortunate we caught the problem relatively early; in cases where memory loss lasts for more than 18 months, full function often doesn't return even after treatment.

Fatigue and Depression

Susan was a kind woman under my care for chronic fatigue syndrome. The most prominent aspect of her illness was a dark, foreboding depression. After she grew to trust me, Susan described how the depression felt in painful detail. She then added she saw no reason to subject others to it, so she put on a "public face" when she was with family and friends. I deeply wanted to cure her, but months went by with no significant progress.

One day Susan mentioned reading that depression was sometimes caused by hypothyroidism. "Thyroid disease was one of the first things I tested for," I said, "but your lab results showed nothing unusual. If you're willing to risk temporary hyperthyroid side effects, though, I can give you a low dose of thyroid hormones to see whether they do any good." Susan agreed; and to my surprise, the medication made a substantial improvement in how she felt. I was also surprised that Susan's next series of blood tests showed no significant change in her thyroid hormone levels.

I ended up increasing Susan's dosage four times before her levels clearly went up; and when they did, they were still within the "normal" range. Susan was a prime example of a patient for whom the numbers didn't tell the whole story.

After a couple of months on the medication, Susan's fatigue and depression entirely lifted. Susan responded by happily throwing away her antidepressant drugs … which had never helped her because they didn't address her real problem, which was hidden hypothyroidism.

Fatigue and Brittle Nails

Jason was a professional flamenco guitarist who normally loved his job, but over the past year had lost his motivation to compose and perform music. He rationalized his lack of energy as career burnout and old age—but he was only in his late 20s!

When I started questioning Jason, he casually mentioned that his fingernails had become a problem. His style of guitar playing depends on long, well-manicured nails. But at around the same time his enthusiasm went downhill, his nails became brittle and kept breaking when picking guitar strings. Jason's manicurist applied increasingly greater levels of protectant, but it didn't help. To be thorough, I tested Jason's zinc and protein levels as well as his thyroid levels. The lab results clearly showed hypothyroidism.

After a year of treatment, Jason's nails were in top shape again. And more importantly, his passion for music and performing had been completely restored.

THYROID FACTOID

Famous people who have had thyroid disease and thrived after treatment include rock star Rod Stewart, movie critic Roger Ebert, comedian Joe Piscopo, Olympic track and field champion Carl Lewis, pro golfer Ben Crenshaw, Nobel Prize–winning doctor Rosalyn Yalow, best-selling author Isaac Asimov, and former President George H. W. Bush and his wife Barbara.

Feeling Unusually Cold

Caroline came to see me in the middle of the summer wearing heavy pants and a very heavy sweater. When we shook hands, I felt that she was freezing. When I mentioned this, she replied, "All offices keep their temperatures much lower than they ought to." She added, "My husband tries to do the same thing at home, but I won't let him."

Caroline was already on thyroid medication, but on a low dosage. I gradually raised it, and after a few months Caroline was dressing normally and enjoying warmth again.

Hair Loss

One of the symptoms that most strongly motivates people to see me without delay is hair loss. Sally was a patient of mine for years, and had been treated successfully for her hypothyroidism. One day Sally came to see me in a panic. She leaned her head forward and showed me the clear thinning of her hair, with lots of scalp showing.

"We need to raise my thyroid medication right away!" Sally said.

"It could be your thyroid," I replied, "but it could be something else. Let me take your blood and have the lab test for the likeliest causes."

The results showed Sally's instincts were right. She tested negative for everything except her previous problem—she'd again become hypothyroid.

I was puzzled, because Sally's condition had been stable for years. I asked if she was taking her medication first thing in the morning, and was waiting 30-60 minutes before eating or drinking anything but water. She assured me she was.

I therefore raised Sally's dosage, expecting her thyroid hormone levels to rise on her next test. A month later, I received another surprise: the levels had gotten even *lower*.

The situation had become so unusual that I decided to question Sally more carefully about her morning routine. This time she mentioned that a few months ago she'd begun taking her thyroid pills with orange juice instead of water. "But that shouldn't make any difference," she added.

"Is it calcium-fortified orange juice?" I asked.

"Yes, it is," she replied.

I shook my head. "Sally, calcium is one of the strongest binders of thyroid hormones. You aren't giving the hormones a chance to get into your bloodstream."

I put Sally back on her original dosage and asked her to take her medication with water only. Sally's blood levels quickly returned to normal, and within a few months over 90 percent of her hair had grown back.

 THROAT QUOTE

How can I control my life when I can't control my hair?
—Anonymous

Hair brings one's self-image into focus.
—Shana Alexander

Infertility

Monica was a 30-year-old who'd tried for years to conceive, with no success. In such cases low progesterone is often the culprit. When I spoke to Monica, however, I learned that she'd been gaining weight over the past few years. She'd chalked it up to "growing older."

I tested Monica's blood, and she turned out to be hypothyroid. This should've been picked up by Monica's gynecologist or fertility specialist, but it never occurred to either of them to check her for thyroid disease.

As it turned out, Monica was quite fertile. Within two months of starting on thyroid medication, she became pregnant. A few years later, my wife and I ran into Monica and her two children—the second was conceived shortly after the first was born. Monica proudly showed off her new family and thanked me exuberantly. My wife mentioned friends of hers who I'd also treated successfully for infertility, adding, "Oh yeah, he gets everybody pregnant!" I was quite embarrassed, but the two of them had a good laugh over it.

Muscle Weakness

Janet was diagnosed with debilitating fibromyalgia syndrome when she was 16. She'd been forced to drop out of school due to her unremitting muscle pain and weakness. She needed her mother's help with such simple things as getting out of bed and dressing. Janet had seen a mob of doctors—rheumatologists, neurologists, and alternative practitioners. They all said her problem was exclusively fibromyalgia syndrome.

Three years later, at age 19, Janet came to see me. The tests I ran showed signs of an old Epstein-Barr viral respiratory infection, thyroid antibodies, and a TSH that was above normal levels. Apparently Janet developed Hashimoto's as a result of her respiratory infection at age 16 … and had been hypothyroid ever since.

After six months of thyroid medication, Janet regained over 80 percent of her muscular strength, and her pain all but disappeared. I prescribed exercises for her to perform to get the rest of the strength back in her arms and legs.

Similar and Overlapping Conditions

If you're experiencing hypothyroid symptoms, you shouldn't hesitate to see a doctor and get your blood tested for TSH, free T4, free T3, and thyroid antibodies. However, that doesn't mean you should skip other types of testing. There are conditions that cause many of the same symptoms as hypothyroidism, and it's possible that your problems are actually stemming from one of them. Further, it's possible that you're suffering from hypothyroidism and some other condition *simultaneously*. Certain conditions not only resemble but frequently coexist with hypothyroidism, making normally unpleasant symptoms even worse.

The rest of this chapter briefly describes common conditions that produce many of the same symptoms as hypothyroidism. If you find one or more of these conditions fits closely with the problems you've having, don't hesitate to bring it up when you speak with your doctor. Take care to clearly explain which symptoms make you suspicious—your doctor will be more interested in what you're feeling and experiencing so she can make her own diagnosis—and then ask if she believes it makes sense to test for some other specific condition *in addition* to your thyroid testing.

Once your illness has been diagnosed, don't stop there; discuss with your doctor whether there are any aspects of your diet, environment, and lifestyle that might have contributed to its development. Dealing with not only your symptoms but the underlying causes vastly increases your chances of achieving optimum health.

Autoimmune Diseases

Hashimoto's is by no means the only common autoimmune disease. Others range from rheumatoid arthritis to lupus to scleroderma. And especially in the early stages, many autoimmune disorders produce the same symptoms, including fatigue, dry skin, and hair loss. So even if you have autoimmune disease, it isn't necessarily Hashimoto's.

Then again, if you *do* have Hashimoto's, that doesn't mean you don't *also* have other autoimmune diseases. Once your body demonstrates a tendency to attack itself in one area, there's a greater chance it'll do so in other areas. It's therefore wise to get tested annually for other autoimmune disorders.

Anemia

If you don't have enough healthy red blood cells distributing oxygen from your lungs to the rest of your body, you'll develop *anemia*. Resulting hypothyroid-like symptoms can include feeling fatigued and weak; mental fogginess; depression; insomnia; developing dry, brittle nails; and feeling cold (especially in the hands and feet). And, like hypothyroidism, women in their 40s and older are especially susceptible.

Anemia is easy to detect via a routine blood test.

Hypoglycemia

Low blood sugar, or *hypoglycemia*, will make you experience hypothyroid-like symptoms such as fatigue, insomnia, depression, and even anxiety. These problems can be severe, but quickly lessen or go away after you eat something to raise your blood sugar.

Hypoglycemia is easy to detect via a routine blood test.

PMS

Premenstrual syndrome (PMS) is estimated to affect over 85 percent of women between the ages of 20 and 40. The symptoms shared with hypothyroidism include fatigue, mental fogginess, memory problems, depression (and/or anxiety), insomnia, lowered interest in sex, and constipation.

Given its monthly cycle, no one's likely to confuse PMS for hypothyroidism. However, the opposite often occurs—that is, ignoring signs of hypothyroidism by attributing them to PMS. It's actually common to have both; and when this happens, hypothyroidism will make a tough time substantially worse. To learn more, see Chapter 17.

CFIDS

Chronic fatigue immunodeficiency syndrome (*CFIDS*) results in fatigue so severe that it's debilitating—lasting for over six months, and forcing you to make major adjustments to your work and lifestyle. In addition to exhaustion, symptoms echoing hypothyroidism include insomnia, memory and concentration problems, weak muscles, and throat pain.

CFIDS is a syndrome, meaning it's a collection of conditions rather than just one disease. So while you might have CFIDS instead of hypothyroidism, it's just as likely that low-level hypothyroidism is one of the conditions contributing to your CFIDS. In the latter case, thyroid medication won't cure you, but it'll definitely help.

Fibromyalgia Syndrome

Fibromyalgia syndrome is essentially CFIDS plus persistent and unexplained muscle pain. The latter is believed to be the result of a malfunction in how the body processes cellular waste—the acids that build up when you exercise.

As with CFIDS, you might have fibromyalgia syndrome instead of hypothyroidism, but it's just as likely that low-level hypothyroidism is one of the conditions contributing to your illness … in which case thyroid medication will help.

Polycystic Ovarian Syndrome

Polycystic ovarian syndrome affects around 5 million women of childbearing age in the United States alone. It shares a number of symptoms with hypothyroidism, including weight gain, fatigue, depression (or anxiety), acne, thinning hair, irregular periods, and infertility.

This syndrome can usually be distinguished from hypothyroidism by its other symptoms, which include facial hair, and one or more ovarian cysts.

Clinical Depression

Standard clinical depression and depression from hypothyroidism are indistinguishable in their effects—they both result in feelings of immense sadness or emptiness, loss of interest in activities that were previously enjoyable, low energy, etc.

The main difference is that the cure for depression from hypothyroidism is quick and easy: thyroid medication, and particularly T3.

However, standard clinical depression is a much longer and more difficult problem to solve. Treatment usually involves talk therapy combined with antidepressants—and, increasingly, T3, even for patients without apparent hypothyroidism. To learn more, see Chapter 16.

THROAT QUOTE

You handle depression in much the same way you handle a tiger ... If depression is creeping up and must be faced, learn something about the nature of the beast. You may escape without a mauling.

—Dr. R. W. Shepherd

Adrenal Gland Disease

You can become hypothyroid even if your thyroid is functioning normally. This paradox stems from a pair of endocrine glands called *adrenals* that your thyroid relies on to be effective. Your adrenal glands produce cortisol, which helps convert T4 into T3. That's a vital function, because it's T3 that does the work of "powering up" your cells. In addition, cortisol gives T3 the ability to penetrate a cell's membrane. Once inside a cell, the T3 charges the cell's storage batteries, called mitochondria, providing your body with the energy it needs.

If your adrenal glands are underperforming, then you probably won't have enough T3; and more importantly, the T3 you have won't be able to do its job because it'll be blocked from penetrating cells. As a result, you'll quickly become hypothyroid. However, your TSH and free T4 levels—which are all many doctors test for—will show that your thyroid is functioning perfectly. This is a prime example of why you should pay more attention to your symptoms than to lab test results.

An additional complication is that because your thyroid and your adrenal glands work together, when one of them underachieves, the other will strain to pick up the slack. If this goes on for a long time, it can result in both your thyroid and adrenals becoming defective. This is another example of why you should pay attention to your symptoms, and seek testing and treatment as soon as you have good reason to suspect a problem. For more information—including how to detect, test for, and treat adrenal gland disease—see Chapter 14.

Pituitary Gland Disease

You can also develop hypothyroidism when your thyroid is functioning normally if your pituitary gland becomes underactive. That's because your thyroid follows the pituitary's orders on how much hormone to produce, and when the pituitary grows weaker, so do its orders.

This condition can be easily picked up by hormone blood tests.

The Least You Need to Know

- Seemingly unrelated symptoms can all be caused by hypothyroidism.
- Hypothyroidism symptoms include fatigue, weight gain, confusion, memory loss, lowered sex drive, depression, brittle nails, dry skin, and thinning hair.
- If you have even one hypothyroidism symptom, get your thyroid tested.
- Talk to your doctor about also testing you for conditions that you might have instead of or in addition to hypothyroidism.

Diagnosing Hypothyroidism

In This Chapter

- Critical blood tests for hypothyroidism
- Other tests you may need
- Obtaining and interpreting your test results
- Why you can't always trust lab ranges

If you're experiencing one or more of the symptoms described in Chapter 6 and believe the cause might be hypothyroidism, you shouldn't hesitate to see a doctor and get tested. The initial phase of this process is straightforward—your doctor takes some of your blood, and then sends it to a lab with instructions on which tests to run. What makes things complicated is that many doctors fail to ask for the right combination of tests; and many doctors also fail to correctly interpret the results.

This chapter guides you through the hypothyroidism testing and analysis process. It tells you the best methods for diagnosing your condition, and explains the most common ways in which doctors get important details wrong.

Some physicians dislike patients learning about diagnostic procedures, claiming "A little knowledge is a dangerous thing." But when it comes to hypothyroidism, it's much more dangerous to be uninformed. After reading this chapter you'll know what errors to keep an eye out for, and how to ensure you're receiving the most accurate diagnosis possible.

Key Blood Tests for Hypothyroidism

The perfect way to detect thyroid disease would be to measure how T3 is affecting the energy levels of your cells' "batteries," called mitochondria. If your mitochondria turned out to be low on power, that would be definitive proof you're hypothyroid.

Unfortunately, medical science currently can't check your energy at the cellular level. So instead of one straightforward test, a doctor who's a thyroid expert will order four indirect tests: TSH, free T4, free T3, and thyroid antibodies. No one of these tests tells the whole story. But if a doctor is experienced at analyzing the results from all of these tests combined—while at the same time paying attention to your symptoms— the chances are great that she'll be able to judge both whether you're hypothyroid and what sort of treatment you need.

> **THYROIDIAN TIP**
>
> If you're already on thyroid medication, or if you're taking some other medication, schedule your doctor's appointment for the morning and delay taking your pills until after your blood's been extracted. This will decrease the chances of medication skewing your test results.

TSH

Your thyroid increases and decreases its hormone production based on the orders it receives from a small organ just above your sinuses called the pituitary gland. When your body is low on energy, your pituitary gland responds by making thyroid stimulating hormone (TSH). As its name indicates, TSH stimulates your thyroid, effectively telling it "We need more power. Get to work and produce more hormones."

Labs can detect the level of TSH in your bloodstream. When your TSH is above normal, it means you have too small an amount of thyroid hormones, and in response your pituitary gland is releasing more TSH than usual to tell your thyroid to step up production. Conversely, if your TSH is below normal, it means you have too great an amount of thyroid hormones, and in response your pituitary gland is releasing less TSH than usual to slow your thyroid's production. In other words, there's an inverse relationship between your TSH and thyroid hormone levels because your pituitary gland is continually trying to address any imbalance.

At first blush, it might seem that the TSH test will tell you everything you need to know. In fact, many doctors mistakenly order this test exclusively to check on your thyroid. But relying on the TSH alone is a serious mistake.

First, the TSH level in your bloodstream isn't a snapshot of your current condition. Instead, it represents a 2-3 month average of your pituitary gland's activities. That's good in that it provides a long-term look at your body. However, it means you can experience hypothyroid symptoms for 2-3 months before your condition is reflected by the TSH test. This can lead to a doctor pronouncing "you're normal" when you're really in the early stages of hypothyroidism.

Further, if you have Hashimoto's disease, you might swing back and forth between hypothyroidism and hyperthyroidism, a condition called Hashitoxicosis. Because the TSH is a long-term average, the two extremes can cancel each other out, resulting in a TSH level that's normal … and that's masking the war occurring between your immune system and your thyroid.

In addition, the TSH level doesn't reflect whether your thyroid hormones are successfully energizing your cells. For example, if you have plenty of T4 but it's not being converted to T3 (see Chapter 1), or if your T3 can't penetrate your cells (see Chapter 14), your TSH level will be normal but you'll actually be hypothyroid.

Then again, you could have a healthy thyroid but an ailing pituitary gland. For example, if your pituitary is underactive, it'll cause your thyroid to underproduce hormones; but the low TSH level will make your doctor think that you have the opposite problem and are hyperthyroid.

So while the TSH test is a very useful tool, it's not enough by itself to evaluate your status.

CRASH GLANDING

You may hear advocates of old-school thyroid methods claim the TSH test is inaccurate. It's true that a doctor relying on the TSH test alone will reach incorrect conclusions for a substantial number of patients. But all this means is your doctor should run a TSH test in conjunction with other key thyroid tests—and while carefully taking into account your symptoms—to paint a complete picture. To abandon TSH testing as old-school disciples recommend would be throwing away one of the most helpful diagnostic tools available for your health.

Free T4 and Free T3

As explained in Chapter 1, roughly 85-90 percent of the hormones made by your thyroid are T4. T4 is a "storage" hormone designed to circulate in your bloodstream, and be stored in your tissues, until thyroid hormone is needed by a particular area of your body. When energy is called for, your body converts T4 to T3. And it's T3 that actually does the work of powering up the mitochondria in your cells.

Labs can easily measure the amount of T4 in your bloodstream that's available for conversion, called *free T4*; and also the amount of circulating T3 that's available for immediate use, called *free T3*.

And unlike the TSH test which reflects a 2-3 month average, the free T4 and free T3 tests reflect the activities of those hormones within the past 7-14 days. These tests therefore offer a more immediate picture of what's happening in your body.

CRASH GLANDING

Your body renders over 96 percent of T3 and over 99 percent of T4 molecules inert by binding them with proteins. (No one knows why, though some speculate it's a way of preserving iodine beyond what can be stored in the thyroid.) However, it's only the unbound, or free, hormones that have any effect on your health. Free T4 and free T3 can't be accurately calculated from total T4/T3, because there are a variety of factors that can affect the totals (ranging from pregnancy to how much protein you've recently eaten) but have zero impact on the free hormones. So be wary of any doctor who runs old-fashioned total T4/T3 tests instead of modern free T4/T3 tests.

Evaluating your TSH level in conjunction with free T4 and free T3 levels provides a much clearer view than can be gotten from considering TSH alone. For example, if you're in the early stages of hypothyroidism, the 2-3 month average represented by your TSH level might not reflect the recent changes in your body; but the more "in the moment" free T4/T3 numbers will show up as low, alerting your doctor to the problem. Catching hypothyroidism early gives you the opportunity to improve your diet, cut down on toxins (see Chapters 18 and 22), and start right away on thyroid medication, which could end up mitigating the severity of the disease; and will definitely make you feel better by eliminating your symptoms.

As another example, if your pituitary gland is underactive, your TSH level will be low, making you appear hyperthyroid. If your free T4/T3 is *also* low, however, an experienced thyroid doctor will know to suspect a pituitary problem and prescribe an ultrasound or MRI to take a close look at that gland.

Then again, your body might be having trouble converting T4 into T3. A frequent cause of this is a lack of selenium, which can be cured by simply eating a Brazil nut a day. If conversion is the issue, your TSH and your free T4 levels will both be normal, but your free T3 level will be low.

The latter is a perfect example of why it's important to test for free T4 *and* free T3. Many doctors are knowledgeable enough to order TSH and free T4 tests, but then neglect to include the free T3 test. These doctors assume that the free T3 level will merely echo the level of free T4. While they'll be correct the majority of the time, in my experience 20-30 percent of hypothyroid patients have a discrepancy between their T4 and T3 levels (that is, proportionally higher T4 than T3, indicating conversion problems). If you happen to be one of those patients, you're at risk of being prescribed the wrong treatment when free T3 testing is skipped.

If your doctor tests your blood for TSH, free T4, and free T3, the results will provide a pretty good view of your thyroid's status. However, there's one other test category needed to complete the picture.

Antibodies

As mentioned previously, the early stages of Hashimoto's disease—which is the cause of roughly 75-85 percent of hypothyroidism cases—can create a condition of Hashitoxicosis in which you're swinging between too little and too much thyroid hormones. The two extremes can cancel each other out, resulting in a TSH level that appears normal. At the same time, your free T4/T3 levels will depend on the state of your Hashitoxicosis over the week before you happen to have your blood taken. In other words, they might be low, or high, or even normal, depending on what stage of the pendulum swing the disease is in.

Therefore, when you're first being diagnosed, the only way to be certain whether or not you have a thyroid autoimmune disease such as Hashimoto's is to test for thyroid antibodies. More specifically, your doctor should test for *thyroid peroxidase* (*TPO*) antibodies and *thyroglobulin* (*Tg*) antibodies. If you have Hashimoto's, the chances are enormous that you'll have high levels of one or both of these antibodies.

Other Testing

Even if your symptoms point strongly to hypothyroidism, you shouldn't hesitate to allow your doctor to test for other causes. It's possible some other disease is actually responsible. And it's just as possible that you're hypothyroid and have another condition occurring at the same time, making your life doubly difficult (as described in Chapter 6).

In addition, you may require examination that goes beyond blood tests. For example, if your doctor suspects you have Hashimoto's disease, he might prescribe an ultrasound to check for evidence of cellular destruction. Alternatively, if during your physical exam your doctor notices a growth on your thyroid, you may require ultrasound testing, and possibly a biopsy, to determine whether the growth is dangerous (see Chapter 13).

No matter what the results from the lab are, always pay attention to your symptoms. If your body is sending you messages and your test results don't reflect them, then the problem is usually with the testing, not with what you're feeling.

Analyzing Your Test Results

A few days after your doctor sends your blood to a lab, the test results—which are usually a small collection of numbers fitting onto a single sheet of paper—will be faxed to her office. As explained in Chapter 4, you can request your doctor's office to fax that same sheet of paper to you. You can then study the results at your leisure before the next visit to your doctor. This will allow you to know what to expect, and to prepare any pertinent questions.

Alternatively, you can request a photocopy of the results after meeting with your doctor. This will give you the opportunity to study the data and more clearly understand how your doctor arrived at her diagnosis.

CRASH GLANDING

Whenever you receive test results, first check to make sure they include your correct name and birthdate. Both labs and doctors' offices handle thousands of patients, and mistakes happen.

Each of your tests will result in a single number that's judged by where it falls within the range considered normal for that particular test. The key thyroid tests and their ranges are as follows:

Key Tests and Ranges for Hypothyroidism

Test name	Typical lab range	Optimal range
TSH	0.4-4.5 mIU/L	0.3-2.0 mIU/L
Free T4	0.8-1.8 ng/dL	1.1-1.8 ng/dL
Free T3	230-420 pg/dL	same as lab
Thyroid Peroxidase (TPO) Antibodies	<35 IU/mL	same as lab
Thyroglobulin (Tg) Antibodies	<20 IU/mL	same as lab

Interpreting results using these ranges is mostly straightforward. For example, if your free T3 level is 300 *pg/dL* (*picograms per deciliter* of blood), then it's normal because it falls within the range of 230-420 pg/dL. Alternatively, if your T3 level is 50 pg/dL, then it's much too low and you're probably hypothyroid.

Similarly, if either of your antibody counts is 900 IU/mL (*international unit for antibodies per milliliter* of blood), then you're way over the normal limit—35 for TPO and 20 for Tg—and probably have an autoimmune disease such as Hashimoto's.

More complicated are TSH and free T4, in which there's a discrepancy between the lab's recommended range and what thyroid experts believe is the actual range for good health. If your results happen to fall into the gray area between these two ranges, then the next section is of vital importance to you.

Why "Normal" Results Might Be Wrong

This chapter previously described how your doctor might pronounce you healthy if he relied on too few blood tests (such as TSH alone, or TSH and free T4 alone). But your doctor might also misdiagnose you as being fine because your results are all in the "normal" range. It's not that the test results are wrong. Labs usually provide highly accurate measurements. The problem is with the ranges used by the labs for what's considered "normal." For TSH, most labs use a broad range of 0.4-4.5 mIU/L (milli-international units per liter of blood). Some labs use an even higher upper limit than 4.5 mIU/L, such as 5.0, 5.5, or a jaw-dropping 6.0.

These ranges were created by averaging the results of numerous people who've been tested. That's a technique that often works; but for reasons that are still being debated, it doesn't work for the TSH test. Based on real-world experience, most thyroid experts consider the real range for TSH to be much narrower.

The American Association of Clinical Endocrinologists (AACE) recommends using a TSH range of 0.3-3.0 mIU/L. And based on my own clinical experience with tens of thousands of thyroid patients, I use an even narrower range of 0.3-2.0 mIU/L. Studies have shown this is the range that results when testing only people who have no thyroid disease (as opposed to lab averages mostly comprised of patients with hypothyroid symptoms). Why shouldn't you be compared to the healthy?

There's a similar, although less extreme, situation for free T4. Most labs use a range of 0.8-1.8 ng/dL (nanograms per deciliter of blood). In my experience, more accurate is the narrower range of 1.1-1.8 ng/dL.

In other words, if a patient with pertinent symptoms has a TSH level a bit above 2.0 mIU/L, and it's coupled with a free T4 level a bit below 1.1 ng/dL, I'll treat that patient for mild hypothyroidism. In the vast majority of cases, the patient will improve within a few weeks of being on thyroid medication. Unfortunately, this scenario is more the exception than the rule. When a lab puts a test result in the "normal" column, most busy doctors will simply accept it, favoring hard numbers over a patient's symptoms.

It's been estimated that tens of millions of people are unknowingly suffering from hypothyroidism. It's bad enough that many of them don't understand the disease sufficiently to identify its symptoms; and worse that many of the ones who seek help are let down by doctors who *also* fail to recognize hypothyroidism symptoms. But it's downright tragic when a patient suspects hypothyroidism, sees a doctor to get tested for it … and is told she's "normal" because her TSH level isn't above the lab's excessive upper range.

THYROIDIAN TIP

Labs lay out their reports by setting results deemed ordinary in plain type, and the results considered to be unusual in boldface or gray highlights. This draws a busy doctor's eye away from anything designated *In Range*. Doctors joke that WNL, or Within Normal Limits, really stands for We Never Looked. But it's a genuinely serious problem if a lab's use of a too-broad range causes your hypothyroidism to be ignored.

Don't let this happen to you. If your test results happen to fall into the gray area between lab ranges and what thyroid experts know to be a more accurate range, discuss the AACE's recommended range of 0.3-3.0 mIU/L—and this book's recommended upper limit of 2.0—with your doctor. If your symptoms persist, and your doctor refuses to treat you with thyroid medication, then use Chapter 4 and Appendix B to find a different doctor.

Analyzing Patient Test Results

Understanding how to analyze your own test results can be easier after examining real-life examples. The following are true stories of people who were tested for hypothyroidism and, thanks to their being given the right combination of tests and the right interpretation of the results, were successfully diagnosed and treated.

For each patient, you'll see the test results first. Try to analyze the numbers, and then read the patient's tale to find out if you've interpreted them correctly.

Memory Problems

Test name	In range	Out of range	Lab range	Optimal range
TSH		24.65 mIU/L	0.4-4.5 mIU/L	0.3-2.0 mIU/L
Free T4		0.5 ng/dL	0.8-1.8 ng/dL	1.1-1.8 ng/dL
Free T3		190 pg/dL	230-420 pg/dL	same as lab
TPO Antibodies		>1,000 IU/mL	<35 IU/mL	same as lab
Tg Antibodies		699 IU/mL	<20 IU/mL	same as lab

Dora came to see me when she was about to flunk out of nursing school. Dora never had academic problems before, but suddenly was finding it impossible to remember what she was reading. She asked if I could recommend any natural memory enhancers. I told her there were lifestyle changes and supplements that could help, but first we should conduct a few simple tests to make sure there were no medical causes for these "out of the blue" symptoms. Dora was skeptical, but agreed to humor me.

I doubted the issue was thyroid disease since Dora's only symptom was poor memory, but I included thyroid tests to be thorough. As you can see from Dora's results, both her free T4 and free T3 were well below their optimal ranges; and her TSH and antibody counts were through the roof. It was a classic advanced case of Hashimoto's disease.

After seeing these numbers I was certain Dora's memory problems would disappear once she was on thyroid medication. However, I warned her it could be several months until the mental damage was fully repaired. Happily, Dora's usual excellent memory returned in only several weeks, and she ended up doing well in all her classes.

Quest for Growth

Test name	In range	Out of range	Lab range	Optimal range
TSH		11.0 mIU/L	0.4-4.5 mIU/L	0.3-2.0 mIU/L
Free T4		0.7 ng/dL	0.8-1.8 ng/dL	1.1-1.8 ng/dL
Free T3		205 pg/dL	230-420 pg/dL	same as lab
TPO Antibodies	11 IU/mL		<35 IU/mL	same as lab
Tg Antibodies	5 IU/mL		<20 IU/mL	same as lab

Bob came to me feeling weak, tired, and with a poor libido. A friend of his was taking growth hormone replacement therapy and feeling great, and Bob believed he needed the same thing. "It's not the right treatment for most adults," I told him, "but let's do some tests before making any conclusions." The results showed Bob to be hypothyroid via his low levels of free T4 and T3, and a high TSH of 11. Ironically, other tests showed Bob's growth hormone level was too high as well! When the pituitary gland makes an excessive amount of TSH, it can accidentally release too much growth hormone at the same time. Thyroid medication soon solved all of these problems.

Weight Gain

Test name	In range	Out of range	Lab range	Optimal range
TSH	1.5 mIU/L		0.4-4.5 mIU/L	0.3-2.0 mIU/L
Free T4	1.3 ng/dL		0.8-1.8 ng/dL	1.1-1.8 ng/dL
Free T3	320 pg/dL		230-420 pg/dL	same as lab
TPO Antibodies		>1,000 IU/mL	<35 IU/mL	same as lab
Tg Antibodies		77 IU/mL	<20 IU/mL	same as lab

Melody couldn't quite put her finger on it, but she hadn't been feeling "right" for the past six months. She was convinced there was some sort of problem with her body. The final straw was her weight slowly creeping up, even though she was a college student majoring in exercise physiology. In addition, she was feeling anxious for no apparent reason. Melody's family doctor had run some basic blood tests—including ones for TSH and free T4—and then told her she was fine. Not believing him, she came to see me.

Medical schools have a tradition of teaching that patients aren't great judges of their health. However, I've learned that most people actually have a pretty good sense of what's going on with their bodies. I ordered a more thorough battery of tests for Melody, including those for antibodies. It turned out her thyroid peroxidase (TPO) antibodies were through the roof, and her thyroglobulin (Tg) antibody count was high, too.

Melody's TSH, free T4, and free T3 were all normal. However, the antibodies indicated major trouble was coming unless something was done. I prescribed a very low daily dose of desiccated thyroid, which helped bind up the antibodies and reduce their harmful effects. (If Melody were not already living a healthy lifestyle, I would've additionally suggested the dietary and toxin avoidance advice given in Chapters 18 and 22.) Over the next few months Melody's antibody levels substantially decreased. She also lost the extra weight, and her anxiety disappeared.

Depressed but "Normal"

Test name	In range	Out of range	Lab range	Optimal range
TSH	3.7 mIU/L		0.4-4.5 mIU/L	0.3-2.0 mIU/L
Free T4	0.9 ng/dL		0.8-1.8 ng/dL	1.1-1.8 ng/dL

Joan was a 43-year-old mother with a full life who began feeling sad for no apparent reason. Soon after that Joan became exhausted performing everyday chores that normally gave her no trouble. Joan's PMS, which was usually mild, grew severe. She noticed her hair was thinning, and she was gaining weight.

Joan went to see her family doctor, who ran TSH and free T4 tests. As you can see, the results were in the lab's "normal" range. Her doctor therefore dismissed Joan's suspicion of thyroid disease and prescribed antidepressants.

Joan felt sure she had a physical problem, so she went to see a different doctor; and then a third doctor. They all told her the same thing: her tests results were "normal."

After Joan gained 30 pounds, a friend of hers recommended me. It took only seconds of looking at her test results to realize Joan was unlucky enough to be in the "gray area" that's within a too-broad lab range but actually outside the optimal range for health.

I told Joan her symptoms were classic for hypothyroidism, and her TSH and free T4 levels indicated she was in the early stages of the disease. After giving Joan a more complete set of tests—which included antibody testing that showed she had Hashimoto's—I put her on thyroid medication. After several months, all of Joan's symptoms disappeared. Joan then focused on losing the weight she'd gained while doctors were telling her she was fine.

Headaches and Back Pain

Test name	In range	Out of range	Lab range	Optimal range
TSH		0.03 mIU/L	0.4-4.5 mIU/L	0.3-2.0 mIU/L
Free T4		0.6 ng/dL	0.8-1.8 ng/dL	1.1-1.8 ng/dL
Free T3		190 pg/dL	230-420 pg/dL	same as lab
TPO Antibodies	28 IU/mL		<35 IU/mL	same as lab
Tg Antibodies	17 IU/mL		<20 IU/mL	same as lab

Tara had an unusual set of symptoms for a young woman: continual severe headaches, debilitating back pain, and painful irritable bowel syndrome. She'd already been tested by an internist, a neurologist, a gastroenterologist, and a rheumatologist, but none of them had provided a credible diagnosis or effective treatment. I looked over all her previous tests and saw she'd never been checked for thyroid disease. I therefore ordered basic thyroid testing, along with detailed tests of her bowel function and an MRI of her back.

As you can see, Tara's TSH level was quite low, which by itself is a sign of hyperthyroidism. However, her free T4 and free T3 levels were also low, which indicated her thyroid gland was underperforming because it was being told to by her pituitary gland. Tara's previous doctors had given her a brain MRI, but it didn't provide a good view of her pituitary. I ordered a new MRI that did … and discovered a growth putting so much pressure on her pituitary gland that it prevented full production of TSH and other pituitary hormones.

A pituitary growth that's benign will usually make the same hormones as the gland, leading to excessive TSH. Since that wasn't happening, I suspected cancer. I recommended prompt surgery to remove and identify the growth. The operation went smoothly—and we were all happy to discover the growth actually *was* benign. Tara's pituitary gland and thyroid quickly returned to normal, so she required no medication; and over the next several months her full health was restored.

The Least You Need to Know

- Your initial hypothyroid testing should consist of TSH, free T4, free T3, and antibody blood tests.
- If you're on medication, get your blood drawn in the morning and then take your pills afterward.
- Have your doctor's office fax over your test results and then use this chapter to analyze them before your next visit.
- If your test results are within a lab's range but outside the optimal range and you still have symptoms, don't let your doctor convince you that you're okay; seek treatment.

Treating Hypothyroidism

In This Chapter

- Choosing the right medication for you
- Mixing medications
- Supplemental non-drug treatments

If you've been successfully diagnosed and your doctor has determined that you're hypothyroid, then you're ready for treatment.

Happily, while hypothyroidism can cause immense suffering until it's addressed, there are few other serious diseases as easy to manage. All you need is thyroid medication, which is inexpensive, relatively harmless, and low maintenance—taking a pill or two when you wake up each morning will typically do the trick.

Further, you have a number of medications to choose from, ranging from natural to synthetic, and from brand name to generic. The key challenge is choosing the medication, or combination of medications, that most fully meet your particular needs.

Desiccated Thyroid

As explained in Chapter 3, the most complete choice for thyroid treatment is desiccated thyroid (also called *glandular thyroid*, natural thyroid, natural desiccated thyroid, or NDT). Desiccated thyroid is made from the thyroid glands of pigs. It's a natural mix of all four thyroid hormones: T4, T3, T2, and T1. Thyroid medications that are synthetic—that is, made entirely from chemicals in labs—contain T4 and/or T3, but not T2 or T1. No one knows if T1 provides any benefits, but T2 has been found to play a role in metabolism and fat burning.

THROAT QUOTE

It should be the function of medicine to help people die young as late in life as possible.

—Ernst Wynder

Another advantage of desiccated thyroid is that it includes significant amounts of thyroglobulin protein, which slows the dissolution of T3. This means one desiccated thyroid pill in the morning is likely to keep you going all day. In contrast, a synthetic version of T3 such as Cytomel will lose its potency after 10 hours, so you'd typically need to take half your dosage in the morning and the other half in the late afternoon—and having to remember to do the latter without fail day after day can become burdensome.

THYROIDIAN TIP

Thyroid medication shouldn't be taken with anything but water. That's because there are numerous foods (ranging from dairy to soy to cabbage to calcium-enriched juice) and other substances (including iron and calcium) that will bind with the thyroid hormones while they're in your stomach, keeping the hormones from moving on to your small intestine and then your bloodstream. You should therefore take your thyroid pill(s) as soon as you wake up in the morning, and wait 30-60 minutes to allow the hormones time to move out of your stomach and into your blood. You can then eat breakfast, and take your vitamins and any other medication.

If you also need a pill during the day (e.g., because you're on twice-a-day synthetic T3), wait three hours after your last meal or snack to take your second dose of thyroid medication.

Another benefit is that if your thyroid is still partially functioning, desiccated thyroid may actually bolster its chances of becoming healthy again. That's because when you consume an animal's gland, the parts of it that aren't digested will be transported by your immune system to the corresponding gland in your body to strengthen it and help rebuild it.

One other positive aspect of desiccated thyroid is its low price. Pigs are raised for their meat—until this medication was developed, pig thyroids were just thrown away—so the cost of the prime ingredient is small. Further, the market is wide open, because no one can patent the gland of an animal that's been on earth for thousands of years. You can typically buy a one-month supply of desiccated thyroid for under

$10. In fact, there's no such thing as a generic version of desiccated thyroid because the brand names are already at generic-level prices.

A potential disadvantage of desiccated thyroid is that the T4:T3 ratio in a pig thyroid is roughly 5:1, while in a human thyroid it's roughly 10:1. In my experience, 90-95 percent of patients do fine on desiccated thyroid's higher level of T3—after all, it's the hormone that does the actual work of powering up your cells, and T4 exists merely to be converted into T3. Further, your body has ways of balancing things out, ranging from breaking down excess T3 into T2 and T1, to converting less of your T4 into T3 and more into reverse T3 (see Chapter 1).

If you prefer to adjust your medication's T4 to T3 ratio, though, you can easily do so by asking your doctor to prescribe a smaller dosage of desiccated thyroid along with an appropriate amount of synthetic T4 such as Synthroid. Your body makes no distinction between the T4 from desiccated thyroid and synthetic T4, so you can freely combine these medications as long as you end up with the right overall dosage.

Along the same lines, desiccated thyroid can be a bit less convenient than Synthroid in that it's not available in as many sizes. If you require a dosage that's not offered by your desiccated thyroid brand, however, you can take a mix of desiccated thyroid and Synthroid to achieve the dosage you need. (Alternatively, you can opt to cut your desiccated thyroid pills in half, as the hormones are evenly distributed throughout each pill.)

A more significant issue for desiccated thyroid is that it's not always available. While synthetic medication can be made in a lab at any time, desiccated thyroid depends on pig thyroids, and occasionally there are shortages of the latter. When this occurs, you may have to call around to different pharmacies to find one with a supply of your medication—or, as a last resort, briefly switch to a synthetic T4/T3 combination such as Synthroid and Cytomel.

Another potential downside is that you may object to the prime ingredient. For example, if your religion forbids you from consuming anything from a pig, or if you're a vegan opposed to ingesting parts of any animal, or if you simply find the idea of getting your medication from a pig yucky, then synthetics may be a better choice for you.

Perhaps the biggest disadvantage of desiccated thyroid is that many mainstream doctors will either be reluctant or will flat-out refuse to prescribe it. There actually *were* issues with desiccated thyroid in the past, but they were solved decades ago (as explained in Chapter 3). In the twenty-first century, desiccated thyroid is the most complete solution to hypothyroidism, and a number of doctors will accept your choice of it if you clearly and tactfully explain why it's your top preference.

Popular brands of desiccated thyroid include Nature-Throid and WesThroid from RLC Labs (RLCLabs.com). These two medications are actually identical, and they're marketed under different names only for historical reasons (see Chapter 3 for details).

Another highly popular brand is Armour Thyroid from Forest Labs (ArmourThyroid.com and FRX.com). This book doesn't mention Armour Thyroid very often simply because its manufacturer had stopped making it, for unknown reasons, while we were writing most of the chapters. Armour is now back on the market, however, and is as excellent as any other natural thyroid medication.

 THROAT QUOTE

The desire to take medicine is perhaps the greatest feature which distinguishes man from animals.

—William Osler

Synthetic T4

By far the most famous thyroid medication is Synthroid, which is synthetic T4, and is made by Abbott (Abbott.com). Synthroid is what most doctors prescribe across the board to manage hypothyroidism. In fact, over the years it's been one of the top 10 most prescribed medications in America.

Synthroid is excellent at what it does—which is provide T4 in a readily available and affordable way, and in a wide range of dosages. The key question you have to consider is whether T4 alone is sufficient for your needs.

As explained in Chapter 1, T4 is a "storage" hormone designed to circulate in your bloodstream and be stored in your tissues. T4 gives your body stability because the hormone is long-lasting, remaining potent for around eight days.

When energy is called for, your body converts T4 to T3. And it's T3 that actually does the work of powering up your cells.

Doctors prescribe Synthroid based on two beliefs:

- Synthroid's T4 will be converted into all the T3 you need.
- T4 and T3 are all you need from your thyroid medication.

These beliefs are often validated. In my experience, roughly two thirds of patients whose thyroids are still functioning—that is, still make a certain amount of T3 and T2—do well on Synthroid alone. (Whether they'd do subtly better on desiccated thyroid is anyone's guess ….)

For roughly one third of patients, however, the T4 provided by Synthroid definitely isn't enough. No one is sure whether it's because these patients have problems fully converting the T4 to T3, or if they simply require direct T3 in addition to direct T4 (which is what a healthy thyroid produces—again, in a roughly 1:10 ratio).

Whatever the reason, if you happen to fall into the latter category, you'll continue experiencing hypothyroid symptoms despite being on Synthroid. In this case you should switch to either desiccated thyroid, or to a mix of Synthroid and Cytomel (to be described shortly).

Synthroid is the best-known T4 medication, but it's not the only one available. Others include:

- Levothroid from Forest Laboratories (FRX.com)

- Levoxyl from King Pharmaceuticals (KingPharm.com)

- Unithroid from Jerome Stevens Pharmaceuticals (Unithroid.com)

There isn't much difference between these brand name versions of T4. The main advantages of Synthroid are that it's readily available from any pharmacy, and sold in a wide range of dosages to fit any need (as detailed in Chapter 3).

Alternatively, you can buy a generic version of T4, called *levothyroxine*, which is produced by multiple manufacturers. A generic version has the same thyroid hormone as any brand name. However, because T4 is minute—much smaller than a grain of salt—it takes up less than 1 percent of a pill. The rest of the pill consists of "filler" material, and your body may absorb one type of filler material better or worse than another, which influences how effectively the T4 will enter your bloodstream.

It doesn't matter if one brand is a little more or less effective at delivering T4 to your body, since your doctor will be tailoring your dosage based on the ultimate effect your medication is having. As long as you keep taking the same brand, and the manufacturer makes no changes to its medication (and your thyroid's status isn't changing), you should do fine at the same dosage month after month.

The issue with generics is that your pharmacy might get in pills from manufacturer X one month and manufacturer Y the next month; and because each manufacturer uses different filler material, one pill might deliver less T4 to your bloodstream than another. If you notice your generic T4 looking different from month to month (meaning the pills are coming from different manufacturers), pay close attention for any signs of your hypothyroidism symptoms returning. If they do, consider switching to a pharmacy that consistently uses the same manufacturer for its generic T4, or switching to a brand name so you always know what you're getting.

That said, as long as you're keeping an eye out for hypothyroidism symptoms, the risk of trying generics is low ... and can save you $10-$30 a month.

THYROIDIAN TIP

If you've been taking the same generic medication month after month, and notice your pharmacy has suddenly given you pills that are a different size and shape, you can perform a quick test to compare them to what you've been used to. Fill two glasses with cold water, and place one of your old pills in the first glass and one of the new pills in the second. After half an hour, check the glasses. If both pills have become equally mushy, you'll probably absorb the new medication just as well as the old one. If you see a lot more hard chunks in the second glass, however, you may need to either switch to a different pharmacy for your generic medication or switch to buying a brand name.

Synthetic T3

If you're taking synthetic T4 such as Synthroid and want to supplement it with T3, but for some reason don't want to take desiccated thyroid, you can instead choose Cytomel from King Pharmaceuticals (www.KingPharm.com).

Cytomel is synthetic T3. It comes in three sizes: 5, 25, and 50 micrograms. You can combine these to achieve any dosage (e.g., if you needed 35 mcg, you'd take one 25 mcg and two 5 mcg pills).

Cytomel should be taken first thing in the morning, along with any other thyroid medication, to avoid mixing it with food. Cytomel loses its potency after about 10 hours, though, so you should ideally split your daily dosage, taking half in the morning and the other half in the late afternoon (waiting at least three hours after eating before taking the second dose).

For reasons that aren't yet fully understood, taking direct T3 such as Cytomel is especially helpful in eliminating depression. That's the case even for patients who don't appear to be hypothyroid—which is why doctors are increasingly prescribing Cytomel as a supplement to antidepressants.

Therefore, if you're exclusively on T4 and still experiencing hypothyroid symptoms, don't hesitate to ask your doctor to add Cytomel to your prescription. Even doctors who are hardcore Synthroid advocates will generally be willing to supplement it with Cytomel.

Alternatively, you can purchase a generic version named *liothyronine*, which is up to three times less expensive. In most cases, the generic will be just as effective as the brand name version. However, as discussed in the previous section, beware of your pharmacy using generics from different manufacturers from month to month, which can create variable results.

On the other side of the expense spectrum, you can purchase a time-released version of synthetic T3 from a compounding pharmacy. This spares you from having to take the medication more than once a day. However, there are serious risks involved (see Chapter 3).

Another downside to compounding pharmacies is that most of them aren't equipped to perform post-production analysis. That's significant, because brand name manufacturers end up rejecting as much as 20 percent of their thyroid pills due to the medication not passing quality control standards. That means as much as one out of five thyroid pills from a compounding pharmacy might have too little or too much thyroid hormone.

Combining T4 and T3

Recognizing that a large number of people do better on a combination of T4 and T3 medication but some have issues with desiccated thyroid, Forest Labs offers a Kosher and vegan-friendly synthetic alternative named Thyrolar. However, the manufacturer missed several opportunities to make this product stand out from the crowd.

For example, Forest Labs could've made Thyrolar's T4:T3 mix similar to the 10:1 ratio of a human thyroid. Instead, it chose a ratio of 4:1 (which is close to the 5:1 ratio of its natural product Armour Thyroid).

In addition, one of the main advantages of a synthetic product is that it can be created from chemicals that are always available. But Thyrolar has had a spotty record of availability, and at the time this book is being written isn't even on the market.

Meanwhile, Synthroid and Cytomel—as well as their generic versions—are readily available; and you can combine them in any T4 to T3 ratio that suits your needs. So the only clear advantage of Thyrolar is that it provides a synthetic combination of T4 and T3 in a single pill.

Arguably, an ideal synthetic thyroid medication would mix T4 and T3 in a 10:1 ratio, include small amounts of T2 and T1, and always be available for purchase. But no such product currently exists; and considering the costs for a new drug seeking FDA approval is $300-$500 million, such a product is unlikely to appear anytime soon.

Meanwhile, the medication closest to this ideal is a mix of desiccated thyroid and synthetic T4.

For example, a 55-year-old patient of mine named Marti had been stable for several years on a 90 milligram (mg) dose of Nature-Throid. While going through a divorce, Marti came to see me about persistent anxiety. Her anxiousness wasn't unusual under the circumstances, so we mostly focused on lifestyle changes to reduce stress. For safety's sake, though, I took some of Marti's blood for testing.

The results showed Marti's cortisol levels had gone up, which is something that can happen in response to acute stress. Cortisol can initially speed the conversion of T4 into T3 (though over time it'll block T3 from accessing cells, leading to hypothyroidism—see Chapter 14). Since Marti was getting too much T3, but I didn't want to lower her T4, I adjusted her medication from 90 mg of Nature-Throid to a mix of 30 mg of Nature-Throid and 88 micrograms (mcg) of levothyroxine (generic T4). After a couple of months, Marti's anxiety faded away.

According to a 2003 survey by thyroid health advocate Mary Shomon, over half of thyroid patients are unsatisfied with their treatment. Some are never given the best medication for them. Others start out well, but grow worse as their medication fails to keep up with their changing conditions. Yet others are on the right medication but the wrong dosage (see Chapter 9).

You should never settle for less than optimal treatment. If your symptoms continue while on one type of medication, insist that your doctor let you try something else. And if your symptoms go away but then recur, or you experience new symptoms, don't hesitate to return to your doctor for retesting.

With all the options available for treating hypothyroidism, you should be able to lead a life just as rich and symptom free as that of anyone with a perfectly healthy thyroid.

Beyond Medication

Thyroid medication is the primary remedy for hypothyroidism, but it's not the only one. For example, if your diet is low on iodine, you're depriving your thyroid of the fundamental chemical it needs to make its hormones. This is especially common during pregnancy, when the body's need for iodine abruptly increases. If you suspect you're iodine deficient, try gently increasing your iodine intake and see if that helps.

Alternatively, if you've been consuming too much iodine—for example, by eating a lot of seafood, or via products with iodine megadoses—your thyroid can respond by shutting down to prevent severe hyperthyroidism. In this case, cut way back on iodine and give your body a couple of weeks to flush out the excess.

THYROIDIAN TIP

If you aren't sure whether you have the right amount of iodine, you can check by collecting your urine for 24 hours and having your doctor's office submit it to a lab. (This is *not* to be confused with the dangerous 50 milligram Iodoral process warned against in Chapter 3; you don't take any iodine for this test other than what you normally consume.) The typical cost is $60-$130; ask your doctor for details.

Then again, you may be low on selenium, which is a key chemical your body uses to convert T4 to T3 (see Chapter 1).

The simple solution is to eat a single Brazil nut daily, as this nut is the richest food source of selenium. (Don't eat more than one a day regularly, though, or you'll end up overdosing.)

THYROIDIAN TIP

If you aren't sure whether you have enough selenium, you can check via a *red blood cell element test*. This is a highly informative blood test that measures your 3-month average levels of essential chemicals boron, chromium, calcium, copper, iron, magnesium, manganese, molybdenum, phosphorus, potassium, selenium, vanadium, and zinc; and in addition detects the presence of the toxins arsenic, cadmium, lead, mercury, and thallium. (For more on toxins, see Chapters 18 and 22.) The test costs around $250.

Something else worth exploring is the traditional Ayurvedic herb *ashwagandha* (Latin name *withania somnifera*), which can help heal and strengthen glands. Ashwagandha is Sanskrit for "smells like a horse," but in its commercial form its odor is typically neither strong nor unpleasant. Ashwagandha has virtually no side effects, so there's little harm in giving it a try.

It's also important to eat foods that foster both your thyroid's health and your overall health. Much more about this appears in Chapter 18.

One other approach that involves zero medicine is a yoga posture called the shoulder stand. It involves lying flat on your back, letting your body rest on your shoulders and the back of your neck, and raising your legs together until they're pointing straight up. It's a little like doing a headstand, but instead of the top of your head you're using the back of your neck, with your chin pressed hard against your chest. This places substantial compression on your thyroid and can increase the blood supply to it.

If any of these remedies help you, then you may end up with a healthier thyroid that's less dependent on medication.

The Least You Need to Know

- If you want a medication that includes all four thyroid hormones, choose desiccated thyroid such as Nature-Throid.
- If you want the bestselling thyroid medication on the market, choose Synthroid, which is synthetic T4.
- If you pick Synthroid, seriously consider supplementing it with Cytomel, which is synthetic T3.
- You can freely mix T4 and T3 medications to achieve the treatment that's ideal for your needs.
- Additional ways to treat hypothyroidism include adjusting your iodine and selenium levels, using the herb ashwagandha, and yoga.

Setting Your Dosage

In This Chapter

- The trial-and-error process
- Avoiding extreme dosages
- Converting dosages among different thyroid medications
- True tales of underdosing and overdosing
- Taking your medication without fail

Chapter 8 helped you choose your thyroid medication. Your final step to health is deciding precisely how much medication you need. If you don't take enough medication, you'll continue having hypothyroidism symptoms. But if you take too much medication, you'll become hyperthyroid, which is a much more dangerous illness (see Chapter 10).

This chapter explains what you need to know to avoid undesirable extremes and arrive at the dosage that's perfect for you.

Finding Your Perfect Dosage

Discovering precisely the right amount of thyroid medication you need is a process of educated guesswork and trial and error, with your symptoms and blood tests as ways of continually checking on whether a particular choice is closer to or further from your optimal dosage.

The first factor to consider is your weight. A very rough rule of thumb is that your body needs one microgram (mcg) of T4, or its equivalent, per pound (up to 300 pounds). That means an adult weighing 200 pounds will need roughly 175-225 mcg of total thyroid hormones, while an adult weighing 150 pounds will need roughly 125-175 mcg.

The other key factor is how much help your thyroid actually needs. For example, if you're in the early stages of thyroid disease, you might require just a little bit of medication to make up for your thyroid's moderate underactivity. However, your doctor may have to gradually increase your dosage over time if your thyroid grows progressively worse.

As another example, if your hypothyroidism is due to external factors—such as a toxin interfering with your thyroid's functioning, or a lack of iodine or selenium— your doctor might prescribe a substantial amount of thyroid medication at first, but taper it down as the cause of the problem is resolved.

Then again, if your thyroid has entirely stopped working, or has been surgically removed, your medication will need to take the place of *all* the hormones a thyroid normally supplies. The good news is there isn't much of a practical difference between being on lower or higher dose pills—they typically cost the same, are around the same size, and have the same rules (take them first thing in the morning with nothing but water). There's even a distinct advantage to fully replacing a shut down or missing thyroid with medication, which is that once you determine the dosage that's right for you, it's unlikely to change. This means unless you notice symptoms returning—or new symptoms—you won't need to have your thyroid hormone levels checked more than once a year.

You and your doctor can determine to what extent your thyroid needs help via two diagnostic tools: your thyroid blood tests (see Chapter 7) and your symptoms (see Chapter 6).

After studying the results of your initial blood tests, your doctor will prescribe her best guess for an appropriate dosage. She'll err on the low side, because there's no danger to your being slightly hypothyroid, while there *are* serious hazards associated with long-term hyperthyroidism, including heart damage and bone loss. For this reason your doctor will ask you to be alert for hyperthyroidism symptoms, such as a rapidly beating heart, acute anxiety, or simply feeling like you drank a pot of coffee when you didn't.

It can take up to three months for your medication to clearly show up as a new TSH level in your bloodstream. However, in half that time your new free T4 and free T3 levels will have stabilized, and your TSH level may at least have started shifting; so to ensure you aren't seriously over or under your therapeutic level, your doctor will typically ask you to come back in around six weeks.

Shortly before your second visit, pay attention to your body while skimming through Chapter 2. If you notice any symptoms that you reasonably believe might be caused by either hypothyroidism or hyperthyroidism, jot them down, and be prepared to describe them when your doctor asks how you feel. If your doctor is a good one, she'll take your symptoms into account along with her physical examination and the results of your second round of blood tests. She'll then use all this information to fine-tune your dosage.

THYROIDIAN TIP

It's common to need a bit less medication but feel as if you need a bit more, and vice versa. But if you changed your dosage on your own, you'd be making a small problem into a bigger one. Instead, simply rely on your feeling that *something* is wrong, and see your doctor for another round of blood tests. The combination of symptoms, a brief physical exam, and lab results will provide a clear view of the current state of your hypothyroidism.

If the change to your dosage is smaller than what you expected, be aware that these corrections are akin to steering a big ship. If you turn a ship's wheel too drastically, you'll soon end up off course. Similarly, when your lab numbers are close to where they should be, doctors prefer gentle and gradual modifications that yield significant results over a month or two.

After your second visit, your doctor will probably ask to see you again in three months, this time allowing for your TSH level to fully reflect your latest dosage change.

If your dosage requires only minor adjustments after your third visit, your doctor will probably ask to see you again in six months or, if your condition appears stable, in a year.

No matter when your next visit is scheduled, you should never hesitate to make an earlier appointment if you notice symptoms returning or getting worse, or new symptoms appearing. Aside from any risks involved, there's no good reason for you to spend weeks feeling awful when a simple modification of your dosage can restore your good health.

Be Goldilocks

Most doctors beware extremes in either direction, and you should, too—even when they come from your own physician. For example, if a man weighs 180 pounds and his thyroid has shut down, and he's prescribed 50 mcg of Synthroid, that's way too low for even a conservative initial dosage. Similarly, if you're feeling awful for over three months on an exceptionally low dosage and your doctor tells you to be patient, find another doctor.

As another example, if your practitioner tells you to take more than three grains of Nature-Throid—the equivalent of 300 mcg of Synthroid—that's flat-out dangerous (aside from rare circumstances, such as a patient weighing well over 300 pounds). If you went along, it would plunge you into hyperthyroidism and put you at risk of a heart attack.

Some alternative medicine practitioners rely solely on symptoms and basal temperature (see Chapter 3) and may prescribe daily doses of four grains, five grains, six grains, and more of desiccated thyroid.

Overdosing makes many people feel awful, but some patients become accustomed to the overstimulation. Periodically I'll see a patient who's on more than three grains of medication who tells me he feels great. I'll respond, "You might feel great on cocaine too. That doesn't mean it's good for you." A stimulant is making your body become more active than is normal, and by definition that's not sustainable. At some point a crash is inevitable.

My first step with such a patient is to taper him off the overdosing as quickly as possible without shocking his system. Sometimes patients come to me too late, however. In as little as six months, serious damage may be done to the heart and bones; plus it's not unusual for such a patient to enter into a permanent state of hyperthyroidism such as Graves' disease.

Don't let this happen to you. Like Goldilocks, steer clear of too little and too much, and stay focused on finding the dosage that's just right for your body's needs.

Mixing and Switching Thyroid Medications

As Chapter 8 explained, you have a variety of thyroid medications to choose from and you can mix these thyroid medications however you like to achieve the type of dosage you desire. That's because your body makes no distinctions between synthetic and natural hormones, or between brand name and generic hormones.

Along the same lines, you can freely switch from one medication to another, as long as you choose the equivalent dosage. If you encounter any transition issues, they'll typically be because over 99 percent of any thyroid hormone pill consists of inactive filler material, and you may find some fillers make it easier for your body to absorb the active hormones in pills than others (see Chapter 3).

You can see which dosage of thyroid medication is equivalent to the dosage of another medication using the following table.

Thyroid Medication Conversion Guide

T4: Synthroid/ Levothyroxine	T3: Cytomel/ Liothyronine	WesThroid/ Nature-Throid	Armour	Thyrolar (T4/T3 mcg)
25 mcg	6.25 mcg	16.25 mg ¼ grain	15 mg ¼ grain	12.5/3.1 ¼ grain
50 mcg	12.5 mcg	32.5 mg ½ grain	30 mg ½ grain	25/6.25 ½ grain
100 mcg	25 mcg	65 mg 1 grain	60 mg 1 grain	50/12.5 1 grain
200 mcg	50 mcg	130 mg 2 grains	120 mg 2 grains	100/25 2 grains
300 mcg	75 mcg	195 mg 3 grains	180 mg 3 grains	150/37.5 3 grains

Please note the following details about the Conversion Guide:

- Mcg = micrograms; mg = milligrams (1 mg = 1,000 mcg); grain = 65 mg for Nature-Throid/WesThroid, 60 mg for Armour Thyroid.

- Thyrolar = synthetic T4/T3 mix, represented in both mcg and grains (it's often sold as a desiccated thyroid substitute). For example, 12.5 mcg of T4 and 3.1 mcg of T3 = ¼ grain.

- Nature-Throid and WesThroid are identical medications (see Chapter 3).

- There's a slight dosage difference between Nature-Throid/WesThroid (1 grain = 65 mg) and Armour Thyroid (1 grain of = 60 mg).

- All medications are available as pills in the precise dosages listed *except* for Cytomel (and its generic equivalent liothyronine), which is sold only in 5 mcg, 25 mcg, and 50 mcg dosages. You can create other dosages by cutting and/or combining Cytomel pills.

- T3 is roughly four times as potent as T4—for example, 25 mcg of Cytomel = 100 mcg of Synthroid.

You should be aware that 2 + 2 = 5 when it comes to desiccated thyroid. For example, a 65 mg (1 grain) pill of Nature-Throid contains 38 mcg of T4 and 9 mcg of T3. Given that T3 is about four times as potent as T4, that works out to 74 mcg (38 mcg + 36 mcg) of T4. However, the Conversion Guide shows that a 65 mg pill of Nature-Throid is actually equivalent to a 100 mcg pill of T4. This fact comes from doctors who have decades of experience with patients switching between thyroid medications, and you'll find the same information in virtually any other conversion guide (for example, see the guide from RLC Labs at Nature-Throid.com/conversionChart.asp).

You might reasonably ask where the extra 26 mcg is coming from. The truth is, no one really knows. However, experts suspect that the T2 and T1 in desiccated thyroid account for its "hidden" extra power.

It's important to be aware of this discrepancy between desiccated thyroid's stated active ingredients and its actual potency. If your doctor isn't experienced with desiccated thyroid, he might look at only the active ingredients and prescribe too much for you. You should therefore always refer to the Conversion Guide when switching between medications … and, if necessary, bring it to your doctor's attention.

Real Patient Dosage Stories

It can be easier to understand the process of selecting the right dosage within the context of people's lives. The following are true stories of patients who required medication for their hypothyroidism. They were all restored to full health once they stabilized on the right dosage.

Total Thyroid Hormone Replacement

Dan had a perfectly functioning thyroid. Unfortunately, it developed cancer. To eradicate the disease, it was necessary to surgically remove the thyroid.

I normally ease a patient onto medication gradually. This wasn't appropriate in Dan's case, however, because we needed to entirely replace the hormones previously produced by his otherwise healthy thyroid.

Dan weighed 200 pounds, so my initial guess was that he needed the equivalent of 200 mcg of T4 daily. The ways Dan could've received this dosage include:

- **Synthetic T4:** 200 mcg Synthroid pill, or 200 mcg levothyroxine (generic T4) pill.

- **Synthetic T4 and T3 mix:** 100 mcg Synthroid pill and 25 mcg Cytomel pill; or 100 mcg levothyroxine (generic T4) pill and 25 mcg liothyronine (generic T3) pill; or a 2 grain pill of Thyrolar.

- **Natural T4, T3, T2, and T1:** Desiccated thyroid via a 130 mg (2 grain) Nature-Throid or WesThroid pill; or a 120 mg (2 grain) Armour Thyroid pill.

Because the only way for Dan to get both a normal amount of T2 and a time-released version of T3 was via desiccated thyroid, I suggested a 130 mg (2 grain) pill of Nature-Throid daily. Dan agreed. Subsequent months of testing—and lack of symptoms—showed that this was just the right medication and dosage for him.

Underdose for Depression

Lori's problem was depression. She'd tried four major antidepressants, but none of them worked for her. When Lori came to me for help, she mentioned that she'd been taking 75 mcg of Synthroid for the past five years. That's a small amount for most adults, so I immediately suspected underdosing as the source of Lori's ills.

Blood tests confirmed this; Lori's TSH was high and her hormone levels below normal. I raised her prescription to 100 mcg of Synthroid, and asked Lori to come in for another round of testing in three months. I also told her to come in right away if she noticed any signs of hyperthyroidism, such as her heart rate increasing.

Three months later, Lori's depression had largely lifted. However, she was now complaining of fatigue. When I questioned her, it turned out that once Lori had started feeling better, she'd begun training for a marathon—on top of taking a full load of courses for a Master's degree! When the lab results came in, they showed Lori's TSH and thyroid hormone levels were now perfect. I explained to Lori that it was simply her newfound enthusiasm for life that was wearing her out. Once Lori adjusted to being healthy again, she was fine on the 100 mcg dosage.

Overdose for Fatigue

Josie was feeling severely fatigued. She first saw a doctor who followed the principles of Broda Barnes (see Chapter 3). Using only the basal temperature test, he diagnosed her as hypothyroid and prescribed a 120 mg (2 grain) pill of Armour Thyroid. When these had no effect, he progressively raised her dosage, reasoning that her symptoms would be resolved once Josie had enough thyroid hormones.

When Josie was up to 240 mg (4 grains) of Armour Thyroid daily, her heart was pounding in her chest and she was periodically fainting. At that point she came to see me for a second opinion.

I first told Josie that we needed to immediately taper her off the extreme overdose she'd been prescribed. I added that since she was feeling just as much fatigue as before, there was a good chance her problem was never caused by her thyroid at all.

I took Josie's blood and ordered a series of tests. A few days later the results showed Josie was in the late stages of Addison's disease (see Chapter 14).

I helped wean Josie completely off her thyroid medication, and placed her on medication that directly addressed her adrenal disease. After six months, Josie was feeling enormously better.

A Dog's Tale

Margy was doing fine on her thyroid medication, so I was surprised to get a panicked call from her toward the end of a warm summer day. All my nurse told me was there'd been an overdose.

"Hello, Margy," I said. "Are you okay?"

"I'm fine," she said. "But I keep my Armour pills by the bed, and my dog knocked the bottle over while I was away at work and ate them all. There was a two-week supply in there! I'm afraid he's going to die!"

I shook my head. "It's probably the mild pig smell that attracted him. This happens from time to time."

"He's running around chasing his tail! Should I rush him to the emergency room?"

"It would do no harm to have him checked by your vet," I said, "but he'll probably be fine. Dogs use a lot more thyroid hormone per pound than people. The most important thing you can do is put the pills where he can't get at them in the future."

"Like where?" Margy asked.

"You can store them in the freezer," I said. "Not only will it prevent your dog from accessing the pills, it'll end their mild odor, so he won't even be interested in them when you take them out in the morning. It's probably the warm summer day—which caused some of the pills' molecules to drift into the air—that made him go after them in the first place."

If you have children at home, similar advice applies—always keep your thyroid medication in a safe place where no one can reach them but you. All the reasons for you to avoid an overdose—risk of heart damage, your thyroid shutting down, etc.—go double for young ones.

Staying on Your Medication

After meeting all the challenges involved with hypothyroidism—identifying the disease, getting the right tests done, interpreting the lab results correctly, choosing the appropriate medication, and determining the perfect dosage—you'd think that patients would take their pills without fail every morning.

Oddly enough, though, some don't. Once their symptoms have gone away, and their pills run out but nothing terrible immediately happens, a certain number of patients fail to renew their medication because they feel like they've been "cured."

In fact, hypothyroidism is usually a long-term disease, and within anywhere from a week to a couple of months of no treatment its symptoms will return. This can happen so slowly and subtly that it's not immediately obvious. Making matters worse is that one of the symptoms is often a slowing of mental faculties that affects judgment. As a result, someone can be suffering for quite a while before realizing what's happening.

You should therefore virtually never go off your medication unless your doctor tells you it's okay to do so. The only exception is if you're experiencing symptoms of hyperthyroidism; and in this case, you should call your doctor immediately to get advice and make an appointment.

As long as you stay on your medication, pay close attention to your body for hypo-thyroidism symptoms, and see your doctor for a physical exam and blood tests at least once a year, you should be able to live as rich and healthy a life as anyone with a perfectly functioning thyroid.

The Least You Need to Know

- Your thyroid medication dosage is determined by the degree of your thyroid's inactivity and your weight.
- Don't hesitate to mix thyroid medications to achieve the exact type and dosage of medicine you need.
- If your hypothyroidism symptoms return, or you notice new symptoms, see your doctor for a new round of tests.
- Keep taking your thyroid medication first thing every morning unless your doctor tells you otherwise.

Hyperthyroidism

In this part we focus on hyperthyroidism, which can make you feel as if you're perpetually drinking a big pot of black coffee. We first describe the symptoms, which include a racing heart, anxiety, and tremors. We then describe other diseases that have effects similar to hyperthyroidism and could be the actual cause of your problems.

Chapter 11 explains the key thyroid blood tests you need, and details how to obtain and analyze your lab results. And Chapter 12 helps you choose among your treatment options.

Hyperthyroidism Symptoms

In This Chapter

- Signs that you're hyperthyroid
- Causes and effects of Graves' disease
- Plummer's disease's rogue nodules
- Becoming hyperthyroid from iodine

If your heart is racing, you're feeling anxious, you're losing weight for no apparent reason, or you're experiencing any of dozens of other symptoms, you may be *hyperthyroid.*

Over 90,000 Americans every year are diagnosed with hyperthyroidism, and millions of people suffer from it worldwide. It strikes over five times as many women as men, and the odds of becoming hyperthyroid increase with age.

In addition to those genetically disposed to the disease, hyperthyroidism is an ever-present danger for the tens of millions of people being treated for hypothyroidism. That's because your body reacts the same whether you have an overactive thyroid or consume too much thyroid medication.

This is the first of three chapters providing you with the knowledge you need to meet the various challenges posed by hyperthyroidism. Once you've read these chapters, you'll know whether you should see a doctor; and how to make sure you receive the best testing, diagnosis, and treatment.

Hyperthyroidism Symptoms Checklist

As explained in Chapter 1, your thyroid regulates the energy level of every cell in your body through the production of its hormones. Hyperthyroidism occurs when the levels of those hormones are above normal. In fact, the first part of this disease's name, *hyper*, is Greek for *over* (just as *hyper*active refers to being overly active).

The excess hormones increase the activity of cells throughout your body, which can be so overstimulating that you may feel as if you're perpetually drinking a big pot of black coffee.

Because thyroid hormones affect every cell, in theory an overactive thyroid can result in any of hundreds of symptoms. In general, though, certain symptoms are more likely to occur than others. These frequent clues to hyperthyroidism appear in the checklist that follows.

Take a few minutes to go over the list and check off any symptom that applies to you. If you aren't sure whether you have a particular symptom, find the description of it in Chapter 2 and use the additional information to make your decision.

Hyperthyroidism Symptoms Checklist

- ❏ Severe anxiety and panic attacks
- ❏ Irritability
- ❏ Shakiness, including hand tremors
- ❏ Heart pounding in chest at over 90 beats per minute while at rest
- ❏ A racing mind that makes it difficult to focus
- ❏ Insomnia
- ❏ Losing weight for no apparent reason (or gaining weight due to an abrupt increase in appetite)
- ❏ Feeling overheated
- ❏ Oversweating (especially in the head, hands, and feet)
- ❏ Tingling in the hands and feet
- ❏ Frequent bowel movements and/or a loose stool
- ❏ Menstrual problems
- ❏ A sex drive that's in overdrive
- ❏ Weak muscles
- ❏ Thinning hair

❑ Thyroid growths, called *goiters*

❑ Eyes sensitive to light

❑ A dry, gritty feeling in the eyes

❑ Enlarged, protruding eyes (creating a "bug-eyed" look)

If you have six or more of these common symptoms, there's a strong chance you're hyperthyroid. Get your thyroid checked out—typically via blood tests for TSH, free T4, free T3, and thyroid antibodies—as soon as possible.

If you have two to five of these symptoms, that's still reason enough to get your thyroid tested. Either the results will be positive, putting you on the path to treatment; or negative, which will inform your doctor to explore other potential problem sources.

But even if you have only one of these symptoms and your doctor isn't providing a satisfying explanation for its cause, you should seriously consider getting tested. That's especially true if you're a woman, as you're at over five times greater risk than a man of being struck by hyperthyroidism.

The checklist is by no means comprehensive; you can definitely experience other symptoms. However, the odds are that along with the unlisted symptoms you'll have at least a few of the ones on the checklist—and the latter are all the clues you need to go get tested.

If you're successfully treated, you'll soon experience improvement regarding *all* your hyperthyroidism symptoms.

THYROIDIAN TIP

Some of the symptoms on the checklist apply to both hyperthyroidism and hypothyroidism—for example, insomnia, weak muscles, thinning hair, goiters, menstrual problems, and gaining weight. In each case, the problem stems from different causes but has the same result. Fortunately, all you need to do is see a doctor who'll test your blood for thyroid disease. The lab results will reveal your condition.

Hyperthyroidism Dangers

Some people actually enjoy being hyperthyroid at first. During its initial, milder stages you can become unusually productive, especially at low-level tasks like cleaning out the garage. But at a certain point hyperthyroidism may become not only unpleasant, but horrific.

For example, one of my patients was a photojournalist who risked his life covering wars and taking pictures of soldiers during combat. He told me the anxiety he experienced was so gut-wrenching that he'd felt safer and more comfortable being shot at on battlefields than he did sitting at home with his family during hyperthyroid-induced panic attacks.

As another example, early on in my career I took thyroid medication I didn't need to understand what my hyperthyroid patients were going through. It was one of the worst experiences of my life. Perhaps it made me a better doctor, but I wouldn't recommend anyone to willingly go through such an ordeal.

In addition to the overt symptoms, hyperthyroidism can cause bone loss (osteoporosis), cardiovascular damage that can lead to a heart attack, and pressure on ocular nerves that can eventually lead to blindness.

In fact, one of the few advantages of hyperthyroidism is that it's not subtle. Especially in its later stages, its symptoms are so severe that most doctors are able to quickly spot them and identify their cause.

Otherwise, as awful as hypothyroidism is, hyperthyroidism is worse. In fact, among the prime cures for hyperthyroidism is turning you hypothyroid instead—typically via drugs, surgery, or radiation that reduces your thyroid's functionality. At that point your condition can be managed via hypothyroid medication.

THROAT QUOTE

It is those who have enough but not too much who are the happiest.

—Peace Pilgrim

Graves' Disease

Roughly 80 percent of hyperthyroidism results from *Graves' disease*. This grim-sounding illness doesn't derive its name from its outcome—it's actually highly treatable—but from an Irish doctor named Robert James Graves who was the first to write about it in detail in 1835.

Graves' disease strikes women about seven times as often as men. It most commonly occurs during early adolescence and ages 20-40, but can happen at any age. Graves' is an *autoimmune* disease. It occurs when your immune system—which normally protects you by attacking foreign invaders such as bacteria and viruses—mistakes your thyroid as a danger and starts attacking it, too.

Graves' is typically caused by a genetic disposition for an autoimmune problem—it runs in families—coupled with a trigger that pushes the immune system over the edge.

That said, most of the triggers for Graves' disease are unknown. The only proven culprit to date is an excess of iodine, the key chemical your thyroid uses to make its hormones. Your thyroid is designed to sift through your blood, and suck in and store even the tiniest amounts of iodine it finds. This ability is normally wonderful, because it means you need to consume only a little bit of iodine daily to have enough T3 and T4. If you have a genetic disposition for Graves', however, your thyroid's sensitivity to iodine may cause your body to identify even a mild overdose as toxic … and as a reason to mobilize your immune system.

Then again, something else can set your immune system on alert—for example, accidentally consuming mercury, which really *is* poisonous, and is so similar to iodine in chemical composition that it'll be absorbed by your thyroid.

Whatever the trigger, your immune system will respond by creating antibodies to flush it from your system. Unfortunately, what often happens if you're predisposed to Graves' is the antibodies will mistake your thyroid cells as being a threat along with whatever triggering chemical they're storing. The antibodies will respond by attacking your entire thyroid; and there's no practical way to stop them. (Your doctor could shut down your immune system, but that would be a "cure" leaving you vulnerable to hundreds of other illnesses.)

As with Hashimoto's disease (see Chapter 5), this may involve *thyroid peroxidase* antibodies and *thyroglobulin* antibodies. But the primary cause of Graves' is *thyroid stimulating immunoglobulin* antibodies, or *TSI*. TSI is unique because at the same time that it's attacking your thyroid's cells, it's stimulating them into producing more hormones.

TSI has essentially the same effect as the *thyroid stimulating hormone*, or *TSH*, secreted by your pituitary gland (see Chapter 1). However, while TSH production is linked to the amount of T3 and T4 in your bloodstream and is designed to maintain balanced thyroid hormone levels, TSI is produced with no regard to your body's thyroid levels, and with no limits. In other words, TSI is like a rogue, insane version of your pituitary gland; and it makes your thyroid produce much more T3 and T4 than your body needs.

The results include all the symptoms of hyperthyroidism previously described— elevated heart rate, panic attacks, tremors, etc. In addition, the extra activity frequently leads to one or more *goiters*, which are enlargements of your thyroid, and to eye problems. If left untreated, Graves' will become progressively more severe. Fortunately, there are a variety of treatment options for this disease (described in Chapter 12).

THYROID FACTOID

Graves' disease has a lot in common with Hashimoto's disease—they're both autoimmune thyroid conditions, and they're both responsible for the vast majority of thyroid disease. The key difference is that the antibodies that cause Hashimoto's attack the inner proteins of the thyroid, which breaks down its cells. In contrast, Graves' is caused by TSI antibodies that attack the thyroid's receptors for TSH—and in the process continually stimulate them. Even after your pituitary gland shuts down in response to your body having too much T3 and T4, the stimulation from the TSI ensures your thyroid will continue to overproduce hormones and keep you hyperthyroid.

Goitrous Hyperthyroidism

A goiter is a non-cancerous swelling on your thyroid. Your thyroid can grow one goiter or multiple goiters. This condition isn't really a disease, but a side effect of diseases such as Graves'.

If you're hyperthyroid, you'll typically develop goiters when TSI antibodies relentlessly stimulate your thyroid to overproduce. Because your thyroid isn't capable of making enough hormones to meet the antibodies' demands at its current size, it grows more cells. This is an effective response when you're healthy, as producing additional T3 and T4 until your bloodstream has a sufficient supply will end your body's requests for these hormones. However, no amount of overproduction will satisfy the limitless demands of the TSI antibodies, which means TSI will make your thyroid keep growing and growing.

If your hyperthyroidism is successfully treated in its early stages with medication, any existing goiters will stop getting bigger, and may even fade away over time. That's because once the TSI stimulation ends, your thyroid will stop replacing dying goiter cells with fresh ones, resulting in natural shrinkage. Alternatively, if your treatment involves surgery or radiation, any goiters can be removed or destroyed as part of the procedure.

Hyperthyroid Eye Disease

If you're hyperthyroid, you're almost certain to have "lid lag." Your doctor can spot this by having you follow her finger as she moves it up and down. If the white part of your eye can be seen above your iris as you look down, it's a strong indication you're hyperthyroid.

If you have Graves' disease, there's also a roughly 30 percent chance that you'll develop more severe eye problems. For example, you can become sensitive to light. You may feel a painful dryness or grittiness in your eyes. Or you may experience double vision (called *diplopia*).

As the disease progresses, your eyelids may retract, and your eyes enlarge and protrude, creating a "bug-eyed" look. If left untreated, this is a serious condition that can put pressure on your optic nerves and eventually lead to blindness. If treatment occurs soon enough, distended eyeballs will return to normal on their own after the disease is under control. Past a certain point of growth, though, surgery may be required.

CRASH GLANDING

If your Graves' eye disease has been brought under control, keep a sharp lookout for any signs of its return. Graves' eye disease can come back, and grow worse, even when all your other hyperthyroidism symptoms are being well managed.

Plummer's Disease

Plummer's disease is the second most common cause of hyperthyroidism. It occurs most often in women, and after age 50. Named after acclaimed American endocrinologist Henry Stanley Plummer (who co-founded the Mayo Clinic), Plummer's disease is caused by one or more non-cancerous thyroid growths, or *nodules*, that produce hormones independently—that is, without waiting to be stimulated by TSH. These nodules are referred to as "toxic" because they churn out hormones at such high levels that they'll make you hyperthyroid.

A single toxic nodule is called *Plummer's adenoma* (adenoma is another name for a non-cancerous growth). Plummer's disease can also take the form of a *toxic multinodular goiter*, in which a number of such nodules spring up on a goiter.

Plummer's disease is typically triggered by insufficient iodine. Specifically, because iodine is the chemical your thyroid needs to make its hormones, a lack of it will lead to low levels of T3 and T4. The thyroid responds by growing more cells in a dysfunctional attempt to make additional hormones—which over time leads to goiters. The goiters then develop smaller growths, called nodules; and these nodules can mutate to produce hormones independently. Once enough iodine is available to make T3 and T4 again, these toxic nodules will turn you hyperthyroid.

Alternatively, though, Plummer's disease can be triggered by an abrupt large amount of iodine. This is covered in the next section.

Iodine-Induced Hyperthyroidism

Taking in an excessive amount of iodine can put you at risk of becoming hyperthyroid. This most commonly happens if you already have thyroid nodules. The iodine overload can transform existing harmless nodules into a "toxic" state in which they produce hormones independently. If the excess iodine is withdrawn, this can be a temporary condition. If you're over 50, though, just one incident can be the trigger for a permanent condition such as Plummer's disease.

For example, a 62-year-old patient named Ricardo came to see me when he was having increasingly frequent bowel movements and very loose stools for no apparent reason. When I checked his pulse, Ricardo's resting heart rate was 100.

Considering Ricardo's age and hyperthyroid symptoms, I asked him if he'd recently had any imaging tests for which he'd been given an injection. He told me that he'd had a CT scan a few months ago that used iodine to help create a clear contrast.

I took Ricardo's blood and ordered hyperthyroidism testing, and also prescribed an ultrasound for his neck. I wasn't surprised when the lab results showed low TSH and high T4 levels. Thyroid antibodies were negative, ruling out Graves' disease. And a single nodule actively producing hormones was visible via the ultrasound, which confirmed my suspicion of Plummer's disease.

Within the first month of treatment, Ricardo's heart rate settled, and his bowel movements returned to normal.

Painful Subacute Thyroiditis

If your thyroid feels inflamed, you may have *painful subacute thyroiditis.* This typically occurs following a respiratory infection—for example, after you've had the mumps, or the flu, or some other virus. If your body's attacks on the virus create high inflammation, that can in turn spawn antibodies that end up attacking your thyroid.

As your thyroid cells are destroyed, the hormones they stored are abruptly released into your bloodstream, making you hyperthyroid. This condition tends to be temporary. However, you should be treated for its symptoms until it goes away on its own.

More information about this disease—as well as other forms of thyroiditis that include stages of hyperthyroidism—appears in Chapter 15.

Hashitoxicosis

Hashitoxicosis stems from Hashimoto's disease, which is an autoimmune disease that attacks your thyroid cells (see Chapter 5). As the cells are destroyed, the hormones they stored are abruptly released into your bloodstream, making you hyperthyroid.

However, this is a temporary state. As the Hashimoto's continues its assault over months, your thyroid will eventually become so damaged that it lapses into a permanent stage of hypothyroidism.

Thyrotoxicosis Factitia

Thyrotoxicosis factitia is a condition in which hyperthyroidism occurs as a result of artificial rather than natural causes. The most typical cause is an overdose of thyroid medication. Taking in too much T4 and/or T3 via pills has the same effect on your body as an overactive thyroid that makes too much of its hormones.

A patient can intentionally overdose in a misguided attempt to lose weight, or to overwhelmingly combat some other hypothyroid symptom. It's also possible to overdose by simply staying on your thyroid medication without sufficiently frequent testing. Sometimes your thyroid will grow healthier with treatment and begin producing higher levels of hormones, which is a good thing; but unless your doctor detects this and decreases your dosage accordingly, you'll end up taking more medication than you need.

> **THYROID FACTOID**
>
> In rare cases, it's possible to consume excess thyroid hormones from meat. There have been at least two outbreaks in which the thyroid tissue in neck muscles were accidentally ground up along with other cow parts for burger patties. These resulted in "hamburger hyperthyroidism" for entire communities.

The simple solution to these situations is to stop taking the excess hormones. The hyperthyroidism symptoms will then usually go away on their own. If the overdosing goes on for months, though, there's a risk of triggering permanent hyperthyroidism.

TSH-Secreting Pituitary Adenoma

Less than 1 percent of hyperthyroidism cases are caused by a condition called *TSH-secreting pituitary adenoma*. As explained in Chapter 1, your thyroid's activities are regulated by your pituitary gland. When your body is running low on energy, your pituitary secretes TSH to tell your thyroid to get to work and make more hormones.

This is a great system when everything is working normally. However, just as your thyroid can grow a toxic nodule, the pituitary gland can develop a non-cancerous growth (an adenoma) that turns rogue and independently produces TSH. In contrast to your pituitary's generating TSH based on your body's needs, the adenoma arbitrarily makes excessive amounts of TSH.

All TSH looks alike to your thyroid, so it'll obey the orders of the adenoma just as fully as the ones from your pituitary gland. Even though your thyroid is healthy, you'll end up with way too much T3 and T4, and become hyperthyroid.

You may also experience other things going wrong. For example, in addition to thyroid hormones, your pituitary gland is responsible for regulating the production of prolactin. Therefore—even if you're a man—you may abruptly start lactating, which normally occurs only in women after childbirth.

The presence of a pituitary adenoma can be picked up by blood tests that show both high TSH and high levels of thyroid hormones. Since TSH and T4/T3 normally have an inverse relationship—when one is high, the other is low, and vice versa—all levels being high indicates an out-of-control pituitary gland whose TSH production is no longer fully connected to your body's needs. The condition can then be confirmed by an MRI of your pituitary gland, which will show an active adenoma growing on it.

If the adenoma is small—under 14 millimeters—it can often be shrunk down until it's harmless via such medications as bromocriptine and cabergoline.

Otherwise, you'll require surgery on your pituitary gland to remove the adenoma. This is especially important because in addition to making you hyperthyroid, continued growth of the adenoma threatens to put pressure on and damage your nearby optic nerves.

Struma Ovarii

In very rare cases—well under 1 percent—a woman may develop an ovarian tumor with thyroid tissue, called *struma*. Thyroid cells don't belong in the ovaries, but sometimes cells grow in inappropriate places. If the struma is distinct enough to not respond to TSH, but similar enough to your thyroid to produce hormones, the excess T3 and T4 will make you hyperthyroid. This condition is treated by surgical removal of the struma.

The Least You Need to Know

- Hyperthyroidism symptoms include anxiety, panic attacks, rapid heartbeat, tremors, weight loss, insomnia, diarrhea, and sensitivity to light.
- Severe dangers of untreated hyperthyroidism include osteoporosis, heart attack, and blindness.

- The most common cause of hyperthyroidism is an autoimmune disorder called Graves' disease, which causes goiters and eye problems.

- The second most common cause of hyperthyroidism is Plummer's disease, which creates nodules that independently produce thyroid hormones.

- Other causes of hyperthyroidism include an autoimmune response to infection, too much thyroid medication, and an overactive pituitary gland.

Diagnosing Hyperthyroidism

In This Chapter

- Conditions with similar or parallel symptoms
- Critical blood tests for hyperthyroidism
- Other tests you may need
- Obtaining and interpreting your test results

If you're experiencing one or more of the symptoms described in Chapter 10 and believe the cause might be hyperthyroidism, you shouldn't hesitate to see a doctor and get tested.

The initial phase of this process is straightforward—your doctor takes some of your blood, and then sends it to a lab with instructions on which tests to run. What makes things a bit complicated is that many doctors fail to ask for the right combination of tests. In addition, some doctors fail to sufficiently consider all possible causes.

This chapter guides you through the hyperthyroidism diagnostic process. It first discusses conditions that resemble hyperthyroidism and might account for your symptoms. It then details the best testing and analysis methods for determining whether you're hyperthyroid.

After reading this chapter you'll know what errors to keep an eye out for, and how to ensure you're receiving the most accurate diagnosis possible.

Similar and Overlapping Conditions

If you're experiencing hyperthyroidism symptoms, you should definitely get thyroid blood tests. However, that doesn't mean you should skip *other* types of testing. There are conditions that cause many of the same symptoms as hypothyroidism, and it's possible that your problems are stemming from one of them. Further, it's possible that you're suffering from hyperthyroidism and some other condition *simultaneously*. Certain conditions not only resemble but frequently coexist with hyperthyroidism, making normally unpleasant symptoms even worse.

The next six sections therefore briefly describe common conditions that produce many of the same symptoms as hyperthyroidism. If you find one or more of these conditions fits closely with the problems you've having, don't hesitate to bring it up when you speak with your doctor. Take care to clearly explain which symptoms make you suspicious—your doctor will be more interested in what you're feeling and experiencing so he can make his own diagnosis—and then ask if he believes it makes sense to test for some other specific condition *in addition* to your thyroid testing.

Further, once your illness has been diagnosed, don't stop there; discuss with your doctor whether there are any aspects of your diet, environment, and lifestyle that might have contributed to its development. Dealing with not only your symptoms but the underlying causes vastly increases your chances of achieving optimum health.

Autoimmune Diseases

Graves' is by no means the only common autoimmune disease. Others range from rheumatoid arthritis to lupus to type 1 diabetes. And especially in the early stages, many autoimmune disorders produce the same symptoms, including anxiety and weight loss. So even if you have autoimmune disease, it isn't necessarily Graves'.

Then again, if you *do* have Graves', that doesn't mean you don't *also* have other autoimmune diseases. Once your body demonstrates a tendency to attack itself in one area, there's a greater chance it'll do so in other areas. It's therefore wise to get tested annually for other autoimmune disorders.

Anxiety

Clinical anxiety is a disorder stemming from problems with brain chemistry. It typically causes many of the same symptoms as hyperthyroidism, including the feeling of being anxious, a rapidly pounding heart, shakiness and tremors, weight loss, insomnia, heated skin, and numbness or tingling in hands and feet.

To discover whether your anxiety originates from your brain or your thyroid, simply have your doctor run thyroid blood tests. If you turn out to have clinical anxiety, it's very treatable via medication and talk therapy. Conversely, if you're hyperthyroid, treatment will make your anxiety fade away … along with symptoms you may not even realize you had until you suddenly feel healthy again.

Irregular Heartbeat

There's a feedback link between your brain and your heart. For example, if you see something threatening, your brain will make your heart beat faster to prepare you for either running or fighting.

What you may not know is that the link goes both ways. If your heart starts beating in an irregular manner, chemicals in your brain will respond by making you feel anxious. Further, in a vicious cycle, your brain will then respond by making your heart beat even faster and you'll end up with all the symptoms associated with anxiety.

This condition can occur due to *atrial fibrillation*, in which your heart's two upper chambers fall out of sync with its two lower chambers, and beat too quickly and erratically. It can also occur due to *mitral valve prolapse*, in which the valve between your left upper chamber and lower chamber doesn't close properly, leading to your heart racing.

If you have such a problem, your doctor may be able to identify it by simply listening to your heart or performing an electrocardiogram (ECG) test in his office. If the problem comes and goes, however, or is a mild case, monitoring for 24 hours or more by experienced cardiologists might be required to spot it.

Adrenal Overactivity

If you have a condition that causes your adrenal glands to produce too much cortisol, such as *Cushing's syndrome* or *pheochromocytoma*, you can experience many of the symptoms of hyperthyroidism, including a rapidly pounding heart, anxiety, shakiness and tremors, weight loss, and bone loss.

For detailed information about adrenal diseases, see Chapter 14.

Bipolar Disorder

The manic side of bipolar disorder can spawn many hyperthyroid symptoms, including abnormal excess energy, racing mind, poor concentration, irritability, anxiety, insomnia, increased sex drive, and weight loss.

If you're bipolar, you're likely to know it; but that doesn't mean you aren't also hyperthyroid. You could have both conditions, with the hyperthyroidism making your manic episodes even more extreme than they would be on their own. The best way to be sure is to simply have your doctor run thyroid blood tests.

Stimulants and Medications

You may be consuming a stimulant or medicine without realizing it's causing hyperthyroidism symptoms. For example, it's common to do more social coffee drinking as you get older. However, your body's ability to break down caffeine *decreases* with age. You may therefore be taking in more caffeine precisely at a time in life when you're least able to tolerate it. The side effects of caffeine overdosing mimic hyperthyroidism: anxiety, panic attacks, irritability, shakiness, racing thoughts, a rapid heartbeat, and insomnia.

Making matters worse, the insomnia can lead you to drink even more coffee the next day to stay awake—leading to increasingly severe hyperthyroidism-like symptoms.

A similar situation exists for other stimulants, including nicotine, weight loss pills, and—on a more extreme scale—illegal drugs such as cocaine and ecstasy.

Some medications also have side effects resembling hyperthyroidism. These include prescription amphetamines, certain allergy pills and decongestants, certain antidepressants, and attention deficit disorder with hyperactivity (ADHD) suppressors such as Adderall and Ritalin. The side effects can include anxiety, panic attacks, tremors, rapid heartbeat, numbness or tingling in the hands and feet, insomnia, diarrhea, increased sex drive, and weight loss.

If you suspect an optional stimulant may be causing your problems, simply stop consuming it for a month or two and see if the symptoms disappear. Alternatively, if you suspect a necessary medication may be the culprit, discuss with your doctor whether you can either use a substitute with less severe side effects or add in other medications that mitigate the side effects.

Key Blood Tests for Hyperthyroidism

The perfect way to detect thyroid disease would be to measure how T3 is affecting the energy levels of your cells' mitochondria (see Chapter 1). If your mitochondria turned out to be supercharged beyond healthy limits, that would be definitive proof you're hyperthyroid.

Unfortunately, medical science currently can't check your energy at the cellular level. So instead of one straightforward test, a doctor who's a thyroid expert will order four types of indirect tests: *TSH, free T4, free T3,* and *antibodies.*

No one of these tests tells the whole story. But if a doctor is experienced at analyzing the results from all of these tests combined, while at the same time pays attention to your symptoms, the chances are great that he'll be able to judge both whether you're hyperthyroid and what sort of treatment you need.

THYROIDIAN TIP

If you're already on thyroid medication, or if you're taking some other medication, schedule your doctor's appointment for the morning and delay taking your pills until after your blood's been extracted. This will decrease the chances of medication skewing your test results.

TSH

As explained in Chapter 1, your thyroid increases and decreases its hormone production based on the orders it receives from a small organ just above your sinuses called the pituitary gland. When your body is low on energy, your pituitary gland responds by making thyroid stimulating hormone, or TSH. This stimulates your thyroid to produce its hormones.

Labs can detect the level of TSH in your bloodstream. When your TSH is below normal, it means your body has too much T4 and T3, and in response your pituitary gland is holding back its TSH to tell your thyroid to slow down or stop production.

Conversely, when your TSH is above normal, it means you don't have enough T4 and T3, and in response your pituitary gland is releasing a large amount of TSH to tell your thyroid to step up production. In other words, there's an inverse relationship between your TSH and thyroid hormone levels because your pituitary gland is continually trying to address any imbalance.

At first blush, it might seem that the TSH test will tell you everything you need to know. In fact, many doctors mistakenly order this test exclusively to check on your thyroid. But relying on the TSH alone is a serious mistake for several reasons.

First, the TSH level in your bloodstream isn't a snapshot of your current condition. Instead, it represents a 2-3 month average of your pituitary gland's activities. That's good in that it provides a long-term look at your body. However, it means you can experience hyperthyroid symptoms for 2-3 months before your condition is reflected by the TSH test. This can lead to a doctor pronouncing you normal when you're really in the early stages of hyperthyroidism.

Further, if you have a back-and-forth condition such as Hashitoxicosis (see Chapter 10), you might swing between hyperthyroidism and hypothyroidism. Because the TSH is a long-term average, the two extremes can cancel each other out, resulting in a TSH level that's normal … and that's masking the war occurring between your immune system and your thyroid.

In addition, the TSH level doesn't reflect whether your thyroid hormones are successfully energizing your cells. For example, if you have an excessive amount of T4 but it's not being converted to T3 (see Chapter 1), or if the T3 can't penetrate your cells (see Chapter 14), your TSH level will indicate you're hyperthyroid but you'll actually be hypothyroid.

Then again, you could have a healthy thyroid but an ailing pituitary gland. For example, if your pituitary has grown a TSH-secreting adenoma (see Chapter 10), it'll cause your thyroid to overproduce hormones; but the high TSH level will make your doctor think that you have the opposite problem and are hypothyroid.

So while the TSH test is a very useful tool, it's not enough by itself to evaluate your status.

Free T4 and Free T3

As explained in Chapter 1, roughly 85-90 percent of the hormones made by your thyroid are T4. T4 is a storage hormone designed to circulate in your bloodstream, and be stored in your tissues, until thyroid hormone is needed by a particular area of your body. When energy is called for, your body converts T4 to T3. And it's T3 that actually does the work of powering up the mitochondria in your cells.

Labs can easily measure the amount of T4 in your bloodstream that's available for conversion, called *free T4*; and also the amount of circulating T3 that's available for immediate use, called *free T3*.

And unlike the TSH test, which reflects a 2-3 month average, the free T4 and free T3 tests reflect the activities of those hormones within the past 7-14 days. These tests therefore offer a more immediate picture of what's happening in your body.

Evaluating your TSH level in conjunction with free T4 and free T3 levels provides a much clearer view than can be gotten from considering TSH alone.

For example, if you're in the early stages of hyperthyroidism, the 2-3 month average represented by your TSH level might not reflect the recent changes in your body, but the free T4/T3 numbers will show up as high, alerting your doctor to the problem. Catching hyperthyroidism early gives you the opportunity to start right away on treatment (see Chapter 12), which is important both in terms of your quality of life (avoiding panic attacks, tremors, etc.) and sparing yourself from the serious damage this disease can cause over time to your heart, bones, and eyes.

As another example, if your pituitary gland is overactive, your TSH level will be high, making you appear hypothyroid. If your free T4/T3 is *also* high, however, an experienced thyroid doctor will know to suspect a pituitary problem and prescribe an ultrasound or MRI to take a close look at that gland.

If your doctor tests your blood for TSH, free T4, and free T3, the results will provide a pretty good view of your thyroid's status. However, there's one other test category needed to complete the picture.

Antibodies

As explained in Chapters 5 and 10, over 80 percent of all thyroid problems are caused by the autoimmune diseases Hashimoto's (for hypothyroidism) and Graves' (for hyperthyroidism).

Hashimoto's occurs when your immune system attacks your thyroid with *thyroid peroxidase (TPO)* antibodies and/or *thyroglobulin (Tg)* antibodies. These antibodies can initially swing you back and forth between hyperthyroidism and hypothyroidism, but ultimately they'll make you hypothyroid.

Graves' occurs when your thyroid is attacked with *thyroid stimulating immunoglobulin*, or *TSI*. The antibodies TPO and Tg may also be involved; but what really matters is the TSI. That's because TPO and Tg attack proteins in your thyroid, and their only effect is to destroy the cells. However, TSI binds with the portion of the cells called *receptors* that receive your pituitary gland's TSH. Very much like TSH, the TSI stimulates the cells to produce more hormones, and this overproduction is what makes you hyperthyroid.

If your doctor runs tests only for TSH, T4, and T3, she won't have enough information to determine whether you have Graves' disease, or Hashimoto's during a hyperthyroid cycle, or some form of hyperthyroidism that isn't autoimmune at all; and such information is vital in choosing the best method for treating you.

Alternatively, if you're in the preliminary stages of Graves', your TSH, T4, and T3 might all be normal; but TSI testing is likely to turn up the presence of the antibodies, providing you and your doctor with an early warning and the opportunity for preemptive treatment. So when you're being evaluated for the first time for possible hyperthyroidism, your doctor should include antibody tests for TPO, Tg, and (especially) TSI.

If the lab results show high levels of TPO and/or Tg antibodies alone, you probably have Hashimoto's and require treatment for hypothyroidism, while if they show high levels of TSI, you have Graves' and require treatment for that particular form of hyperthyroidism.

Other Testing

As the first section of this chapter indicated, even if your symptoms point strongly to hyperthyroidism, you shouldn't hesitate to allow your doctor to test for other causes. It's possible some other disease is actually responsible. And it's just as possible that you're hyperthyroid and have another condition occurring at the same time, making your life doubly difficult.

In addition, you may require examination that goes beyond blood tests. For example, if your doctor wants to confirm that you have Graves' disease, he might request an ultrasound to see whether your thyroid shows signs of enlarging (resulting from TSI overstimulation).

Another common diagnostic tool is an *iodine uptake and thyroid scan*. For this procedure, your doctor injects you with or has you swallow a tiny amount of radioactive iodine, waits 6-24 hours, and then scans your neck to get a clear picture of what's going on inside it. If the resulting images show even, diffuse enlargement of your thyroid, you probably have Graves' disease. If the iodine concentrates in a few areas of your thyroid, that indicates the toxic nodules of Plummer's disease. Then again, if there are areas of your thyroid that don't absorb the iodine at all, that's reason to suspect thyroid cancer, in which case the next step should be a biopsy (see Chapter 13).

No matter what the results from the lab are, always pay attention to your symptoms. If your body is sending you messages and your test results don't reflect them, then the problem is usually with the testing, not with what you're feeling.

Analyzing Your Test Results

A few days after your doctor sends your blood to a lab, the test results—which are usually a small collection of numbers fitting onto a single sheet of paper—will be faxed to her office. As explained in Chapter 4, you can request your doctor's office to fax that same sheet of paper to you. You can then study the results at your leisure before the next visit to your doctor. This will allow you to know what to expect, and to prepare any pertinent questions.

Alternatively, you can request a photocopy of the results after meeting with your doctor. This will give you the opportunity to study the data and more clearly understand how your doctor arrived at her diagnosis.

CRASH GLANDING

Whenever you receive test results, first check to make sure they include your correct name and birth date. Both labs and doctors' offices handle thousands of patients, and mistakes happen.

Each of your tests will result in a single number that's judged by where it falls within the range considered normal for that particular test. The key thyroid tests and their ranges are as follows:

Key Tests and Ranges for Hypothyroidism

Test name	Typical lab range	Optimal range
TSH	0.4-4.5 mIU/L	0.3-2.0 mIU/L
Free T4	0.8-1.8 ng/dL	1.1-1.8 ng/dL
Free T3	230-420 pg/dL	same as lab
Thyroid Peroxidase (TPO) Antibodies	<35 IU/mL	same as lab

continues

Key Tests and Ranges for Hypothyroidism (continued)

Test name	Typical lab range	Optimal range
Thyroglobulin (Tg) Antibodies	<20 IU/mL	same as lab
TSImmunoglobulin (TSI) Antibodies	<125% activity	same as lab

Interpreting results using these ranges is mostly straightforward. For example, if your free T3 level is 300 pg/dL (picograms per deciliter of blood), then it's normal because it falls within the range of 230-420 pg/dL. Alternatively, if your T3 level is 700 pg/dL, then it's much too high and you're probably hyperthyroid.

Similarly, if your TPO antibody count is 900 IU/mL (international unit for antibodies per milliliter of blood), then you're way over the normal limit of 35 IU/mL and probably have an autoimmune disease.

A bit more complicated is the range for TSI antibodies. TSI measures how effectively antibodies in your blood bind to cell receptors in the organ of a lab rodent. This is calculated as a percentage, with anything below 125 percent considered as being within normal range.

"Normal" is misleading in this case, though. If you're at no risk for hyperthyroidism, your TSI score should actually be below 2 percent—that is, at or close to zero. If your level is between 2 percent and 125 percent, it means you might be on the path to Graves' disease. In this case, it's wise to start taking preventive measures to keep your TSI low, such as ensuring you're consuming enough iodine and selenium (see Chapter 1) and are avoiding toxins (see Chapter 22). As long as your TSI level remains below 125 percent, you're unlikely to develop hyperthyroidism symptoms.

THYROIDIAN TIP

When the TSI test reports you have antibodies, it's almost always accurate. When it doesn't, however, there's a 10-20 percent chance your thyroid is being attacked by a form of stimulating antibody that this test just doesn't happen to detect. If your TSI results are under 125 percent but you still suspect you have Graves', you can ask your doctor to focus on other evidence, including low TSH, high T4 and T3, eye problems, and ultrasound and/or thyroid scan tests that show diffuse enlargement of the thyroid.

One other complication with thyroid lab tests is interpreting TSH and free T4 results, because there's a discrepancy between the lab's recommended hypothyroid ranges and what thyroid experts believe is the actual range for good health. If your tests shows you're hyperthyroid, you don't have to worry about this. Otherwise, see Chapter 7 for details.

Analyzing Patient Test Results

Understanding how to analyze your own test results can be easier after examining real-life examples. The following are true stories of people who were tested for hyperthyroidism and, thanks to their being given the right combination of tests and the right interpretation of the results, were successfully diagnosed and treated.

For each patient, you'll see the test results first. Try to analyze the numbers, and then read the patient's tale to find out if you've interpreted them correctly.

Anxiety

Test name	In range	Out of range	Lab range	Optimal range
TSH	0.8 mIU/L		0.4-4.5 mIU/L	0.3-2.0 mIU/L
Free T4		2.9 ng/dL	0.8-1.8 ng/dL	1.1-1.8 ng/dL
Free T3	290 pg/dL		230-420 pg/dL	same as lab
TPO Antibodies	6 IU/mL		<35 IU/mL	same as lab
Tg Antibodies		>1,000 IU/mL	<20 IU/mL	same as lab
TSI Antibodies	0%		<125%	same as lab

Debbie came to see me in a state of frustration. When she turned 40 a year earlier, she was struck out of the blue with severe anxiety. She'd been to four doctors, and none of them offered a satisfying explanation or successful treatment. Each of them simply indicated she must be "wired" for clinical anxiety. "It's ridiculous," Debbie told me. "I'm the most mellow, low-stress person you could imagine."

As we talked, I learned Debbie's older sister also developed anxiety after turning 40. Her sister was diagnosed with Graves' disease, and after it was treated the problem went away.

Each of the previous doctors has tested Debbie's TSH, found it within the normal range, and dismissed thyroid disease as a possible cause. However, none of them had looked beyond TSH.

I ordered a full range of thyroid blood tests for Debbie. As you can see, her TSH was indeed in the normal range. However, her free T4 was elevated and her Tg antibody count was so high that it was off the charts. That meant Debbie was suffering from an autoimmune thyroid disorder.

Debbie tested negative for TSI, which indicated she didn't have Graves' disease. The TSI test can miss antibodies 10-20 percent of the time, but in this case the negative result made sense.

Considering the normal TSH level, I was pretty sure Debbie was suffering from Hashitoxicosis, an early stage of Hashimoto's disease that swings a patient between hyperthyroid and hypothyroid states. Because the TSH level is a three-month average, the extreme highs and lows tend to cancel each other out, resulting in a TSH that appears normal.

I ordered an ultrasound test to confirm my diagnosis. The images of Debbie's thyroid showed precisely the damage I expected from Hashitoxicosis.

I treated Debbie for both the hyperthyroid and hypothyroid aspects of her disease, which eased her anxiety. Eventually Debbie's condition settled into classic hypothyroidism on its own, which was easily treated with thyroid medication.

Lump in the Neck

Test name	In range	Out of range	Lab range	Optimal range
TSH		<0.01 mIU/L	0.4-4.5 mIU/L	0.3-2.0 mIU/L
Free T4		2.4 ng/dL	0.8-1.8 ng/dL	1.1-1.8 ng/dL
Free T3		540 pg/dL	230-420 pg/dL	same as lab
TPO Antibodies	7 IU/mL		<35 IU/mL	same as lab
Tg Antibodies	3 IU/mL		<20 IU/mL	same as lab
TSI Antibodies		158%	<125%	same as lab

Angie had a clearly visible growth in her neck. "It's been there a while," she said. "I didn't come in sooner because I was terrified it's cancer. And I still am, but ignoring it hasn't kept it from growing bigger." I assured her that a lot of people react the same way, and that I'd do my best for her no matter what it was.

I gave Angie a brief physical exam, and found the lump was on her thyroid. I asked Angie if she'd noticed anything else unusual. "I'm embarrassed to say this," she replied, "but over the last six months I've been sweating like a geyser from my hands, feet, underarms, and the back of my head." I ran through a symptoms checklist with her, and discovered that she had a strong appetite but was continually losing weight: "My friends say it looks like I'm wasting away. It's another reason I fear it's cancer."

"Angie, does the lump hurt?" I asked. "Sometimes," she said. "And I'm finding it harder to swallow."

"That's actually good news," I said, "because cancer usually doesn't hurt. And your collection of symptoms make me suspect another cause. Let's run some tests."

As you can see, Angie's TSH was so low it was off the charts. She also had high levels of T4 and T3, and of TSI antibodies. It was a classic case of Graves' disease, complete with goiter.

I prescribed 10 mg daily of Tapazole (see Chapter 12) to manage Angie's hyperthyroidism. That was just enough to make her symptoms tolerable, but not enough to raise her TSH level. Keeping Angie's TSH low discouraged her thyroid from creating new cells for her goiter. Because the current cells died out without being replaced, the goiter shrank naturally over the next year until its size was insignificant.

Angie and I had to continue keeping her TSH low so the goiter wouldn't grow back, but after another year on the Tapazole her Graves' disease petered out, allowing Angie to enjoy normal thyroid function again.

Keeping Her Baby Healthy

Test name	In range	Out of range	Lab range	Optimal range
TSH		<0.01 mIU/L	0.4-4.5 mIU/L	0.3-2.0 mIU/L
Free T4		2.9 ng/dL	0.8-1.8 ng/dL	1.1-1.8 ng/dL
Free T3		500 pg/dL	230-420 pg/dL	same as lab
TPO Antibodies	11 IU/mL		<35 IU/mL	same as lab
Tg Antibodies	2 IU/mL		<20 IU/mL	same as lab
TSI Antibodies		180%	<125%	same as lab

Because of its hormonal upheavals, pregnancy is sometimes the trigger for thyroid autoimmune disease. That's why good obstetricians periodically run blood tests to check for such occurrences. And that's how Sally discovered, near the end of her first trimester, that her TSH level was an off-the-charts <0.01. This meant her pituitary gland had essentially shut down its TSH production.

Sally's obstetrician referred her to me. While I examined Sally, we chatted. "I've been feeling anxious," she said, "and my heart has been beating super fast, but this is my first baby. I just assumed it was all part of being pregnant."

After hearing this, I took Sally's blood and ordered a full range of thyroid tests. As you can see, Sally turned out to have high levels of T4, T3, and TSI antibodies, which meant she had Graves' disease. I followed up with an ultrasound, which confirmed the diagnosis via images of an enlarged thyroid.

I explained to Sally that treatment was especially important in her case because Graves' posed a risk for a miscarriage, birth defects, and heart damage. There was also a risk of the disease spreading to her baby unless we got it under control.

I put Sally on a 2-month starting dose of PTU (see Chapter 12). This lowered Sally's T4 and T3 into the normal range, but her TSI remained at 180 percent. I countered with a gentle increase in the PTU dosage. I was relieved six weeks later when Sally's TSI came down to 75 percent. I kept Sally at the same dosage for the remainder of her pregnancy. She had a beautiful baby boy, with no complications.

Over-the-Counter

Test name	In range	Out of range	Lab range	Optimal range
TSH		0.04 mIU/L	0.4-4.5 mIU/L	0.3-2.0 mIU/L
Free T4		4.2 ng/dL	0.8-1.8 ng/dL	1.1-1.8 ng/dL
Free T3		670 pg/dL	230-420 pg/dL	same as lab
TPO Antibodies	0 IU/mL		<35 IU/mL	same as lab
Tg Antibodies	3 IU/mL		<20 IU/mL	same as lab
TSI Antibodies	1%		<125%	same as lab

Leonard was a charming gentleman in his 60s who loved to talk about diet and supplements, and took dozens of over-the-counter medications.

Leonard came to me because both of his hands had developed tremors over the past year, and the condition was growing worse. While we talked, I learned that Leonard was also experiencing a rapid heartbeat and trouble sleeping.

I ran a battery of tests. The most significant results were his thyroid blood test numbers: a low TSH, and very high T4 and T3.

I remembered Leonard's over-the-counter pills, and asked him to bring them all in for me to examine. One of the bottles was for weight loss, and it listed "lyophilized bovine thyroid extract" as an ingredient. The active hormones of non-prescription supplements are supposed to be removed before they're sold; but these drugs aren't carefully monitored, and accidents happen. Leonard took four of these pills three times daily. Considering he had no antibody activity, I was pretty sure Leonard's over-the-counter meds were behind his hyperthyroidism.

I advised Leonard to stop taking his weight loss pills (which weren't good for him anyway). After four months, Leonard's TSH, T4, and T3 returned to normal, his tremors went away, his heart rate quieted down, and he once again slept soundly.

The Least You Need to Know

- Your initial hyperthyroidism testing should consist of TSH, free T4, free T3, and antibody blood tests.

- Talk to your doctor about also testing for conditions that cause similar symptoms, such as other autoimmune diseases, heart problems, or bad reactions to medication.

- Request a photocopy of your test results, or have your doctor's office fax them, and then use this chapter to analyze them.

- If your TSI score is over 125%, you probably have Graves' disease. Your doctor can verify this via an ultrasound or thyroid scan test. This condition is serious, but highly treatable.

Treating Hyperthyroidism

In This Chapter

- Managing mild hyperthyroidism naturally
- Managing with Tapazole or PTU
- Mixing natural and prescription medications
- Considering radiation and surgery

For those who are hypothyroid, treatment is relatively easy; all that's required are pills supplying the hormones they're missing. Since these are the same hormones normally made by the thyroid, their bodies simply welcome the boost the medication provides.

But if you've been diagnosed as hyperthyroid, you effectively need to combat your body's natural ability to produce thyroid hormones, which is a trickier process. It can be successfully achieved via low-impact remedies, antithyroid medication, radioactive iodine, and/or surgery—and the help of an experienced doctor who carefully monitors your progress.

This chapter will guide you through the options so you can make the best choices for your long-term health.

THROAT QUOTE

For fast-acting relief, try slowing down.

—Lily Tomlin

Low-Impact Remedies

If you get tested as soon as you notice hyperthyroidism symptoms, the disease might be detected at a sufficiently early stage for your excess T4 and T3 levels to be relatively mild. This doesn't occur often with Graves' disease, but it does with other forms of hyperthyroidism such as Plummer's. If you're being treated by a doctor familiar with natural medicine, identifying your condition early on provides an opportunity to try gentle remedies to keep the hyperthyroidism from becoming worse.

The advantages to this approach are that the risks of side effects are near zero, and it'll cost much less than prescription medication. If your condition can be stabilized, you may be able to stay on the non-intrusive treatment until the disease burns itself out over 2-3 years. At the end of this process, your thyroid might return to normal; or you might become hypothyroid, in which case you'd simply start taking thyroid medication (as described in Chapters 8 and 9).

Fluoride

Fluoride is famous for fighting tooth decay. However, it can also combat hyperthyroidism. That's because your thyroid's hormone production is dependent on iodine, and fluoride's chemical composition is so similar to iodine that your thyroid can't tell the difference between the two. Your thyroid will therefore absorb any fluoride in your bloodstream. The more fluoride your thyroid takes in, the less room there is for iodine, and the more likely it is that the fluoride will block iodine from your thyroid's hormone construction sites. The result is a substantial reduction in thyroid hormones.

In fact, some speculate that the current hypothyroidism epidemic is in part due to fluoride being added to the water supply of many communities (see Chapter 22). But what's important for you is that fluoride is an effective suppressor of T4 and T3 overproduction. It's also relatively harmless.

Fluoride was frequently used to treat hyperthyroidism in the past. It isn't anymore, possibly because there's no financial incentive for drug companies to champion its use when there are much more expensive alternatives. But if you can find a doctor who'll agree to monitor its use, you'll discover fluoride can be purchased cheaply from virtually any drugstore; in numerous forms (chewable tablets, gels, lozenges, etc.); and generally causes no complications in moderate dosages, even if you take it daily for several years.

L-Carnitine

Carnitine is an amino acid present in virtually every cell of your body. It's made by your body, and is also present in red meat, diary products, nuts and seeds, and a variety of other foods. Moderately increasing its levels in your bloodstream is likely to have no side effects.

Carnitine's function is to transport fats to your mitochondria so they can transform them into energy. At an appropriate dosage determined by your doctor, though, it has the additional effect of interfering with your T3's ability to penetrate cell membranes, and with your thyroid's responsiveness to TSH. Both of these actions serve to reduce hyperthyroidism.

Carnitine is commercially available under the name *L-carnitine*. It's inexpensive, and can be purchased in multiple forms (tablet, capsule, liquid) from most health food stores.

Goitrogens

Some of the healthiest foods in the world can reduce your T4/T3 count. Cruciferous vegetables such as broccoli, cauliflower, cabbage, Brussels sprouts, and kale are loaded with the compound *indole-3-carbinol*. When eaten in normal amounts, these vegetables are unlikely to impact your thyroid. But if you eat an unusually large quantity of them—more than two cups (100 grams) raw or five cups cooked daily—or if you take indole-3-carbinol in a concentrated form via tablets or capsules, you'll inhibit your thyroid's ability to absorb iodine, and that will result in your thyroid making less of its hormones.

Similarly, soy-based foods such as tofu, tempeh, edamame, yuba, miso, and soy milk are packed with compounds called *isoflavones*. If you consume a lot of soy products— more than two servings (100 grams) of soy food or six ounces of soy milk—or if you take concentrated isoflavones via tablets or capsules, they can stop iodine from being digested properly, which will keep it from entering your bloodstream where it can be absorbed by your thyroid.

These foods are sometimes referred to as *goitrogens* because they have the ability to spur hypothyroidism, which in turn can lead to goiters (see Chapter 5).

If you're hyperthyroid, though, a reduction in T4/T3 levels is a good thing. Since cruciferous vegetables have many other health benefits, including reducing your risk of cancer, and soy products can lower your cholesterol, go ahead and enjoy eating a lot of these foods.

CRASH GLANDING

Other foods touted as reducing thyroid hormone levels include the seaweed *Sargassum,* and the herb *bugleweed (Lycopus virginica).* In my experience, however, these aren't effective for managing hyperthyroidism.

While You're Waiting ...

Low-impact remedies can be very effective, but you have to be patient to experience their effects. That's because your thyroid has already made and stored a large amount of its hormones, and it'll take 4-6 weeks for those existing supplies to be used up. All the remedies can do is reduce the subsequent amount of hormones your thyroid produces. You should therefore allow for 4-6 weeks before noticing a difference in how you feel.

That doesn't mean you need to suffer while you wait, though. You can, and should, take steps to manage your symptoms. You can use prescription medication to do this, and options are described later in this chapter. But natural remedies are available for this purpose as well.

For example, you can typically slow down your heart rate by consuming more magnesium. You can do this in part by eating magnesium-rich foods, such as legumes (adzuki beans, black beans, peas), dark green leafy vegetables (spinach, kale), nuts and seeds (almonds, cashews, pumpkin seeds), and whole grains. Alternatively, or in addition, you can take magnesium in concentrated form via pills.

It also helps to cut down or stop drinking caffeinated beverages, such as soda and coffee, that both reduce magnesium and raise your heart rate.

As another example, if you're experiencing anxiety, you may be able to calm it with theanine, an amino acid commonly present in tea (and one of the reasons people find tea soothing). You might also benefit from kava-kava, a beverage made from the plant of the same name, which relaxes without affecting mental clarity.

As with the antithyroid remedies, the advantages to these symptom dampeners are that they're low-cost, readily available, and have almost no side effects.

Prescription Medications

The primary medication for treating hyperthyroidism is *Tapazole*. There's also a generic version called *methimazole*. A secondary option is *propylthiouracil*, or *PTU*. PTU is an older drug, and it's available as a generic exclusively (i.e., there's no brand name).

Tapazole and PTU are called antithyroid medications because they work by fighting against your thyroid's natural functions. Specifically, they disrupt the process your thyroid uses to turn iodine into hormones. They're very effective at reducing T4 and T3 production, regardless of the form and severity of your hyperthyroidism.

Therefore, if your condition has gotten beyond the early, mild stage described in the previous section, these medications are typically your best choice for managing your hyperthyroidism. Once your condition is stabilized, you can usually stay on them until the disease runs its course over 2-3 years. At that point your thyroid might return to normal; or you might become hypothyroid and simply go on thyroid medication.

Tapazole vs. PTU

Tapazole has several highly significant advantages over PTU:

- It produces results faster, typically returning your hormone levels to normal in 4-6 weeks. PTU may take 3-4 months to do the same thing.

- It needs to be taken only once a day. PTU has to be taken two or three times a day.

- It will have virtually no effect on any subsequent attempt for treatment using radioactive iodine. PTU reduces the odds of subsequent radiation being effective.

- It has fewer serious side effects.

You'd typically turn to PTU if you were allergic to Tapazole or found Tapazole to be ineffective for you. PTU is also preferable for treating Graves' disease during the first trimester of pregnancy, because Tapazole has a greater chance of causing birth defects during the first three months of fetal development. Otherwise, Tapazole is the best treatment choice for most people.

Tapazole and PTU Side Effects

Both Tapazole and PTU share some side effects. When taking either of them, there's up to a 13 percent chance you'll experience itching, rash, hives, joint pain, arthritis, fever, abnormal taste sensations, nausea, or vomiting.

There's also a tiny (0.2-0.5 percent) chance of developing *agranulocytosis*, which causes a reduction in the white blood cells that fight infection—and a very serious chink in the armor of your immune system. Your doctor should periodically test for this. Further, if you get a sore throat or other infection while on either medication, see your doctor right away so she can run a white cell count on your blood; and don't take the medication again until the lab results arrive and show that you're okay.

In addition, PTU has one major side effect that resulted in a 2009 FDA warning: the potential to cause severe liver damage. While this rarely occurs, when it happens it can completely shut down the liver; and it's led to 13 deaths and 11 liver transplants to date. That means if you're on PTU, both you and your doctor need to pay special attention for telltale signs of liver problems, such as a yellowish tinge to the skin or eyes.

Doctors who favor radioactive iodine as a first-line treatment for hyperthyroidism point to PTU's drawbacks, arguing radiation is a more convenient and safer approach. And in this case, a reasonable argument can be made.

When it comes to Tapazole, however, it's been my experience that as long as you have a knowledgeable doctor to monitor you, using this medication creates few complications; and its benefits far outweigh the risks.

THYROIDIAN TIP

Natural versus prescription medication doesn't have to be an either/or choice. Most of my patients do extremely well starting off on low to moderate doses of Tapazole (prescription medication) in combination with fluoride and L-carnitine (low-impact remedies). After a few months, I'm able to wean most of them off the Tapazole, at which point they do fine on the fluoride and L-carnitine alone—which are inexpensive and have virtually no side effects.

Other Medications

While both Tapazole and PTU are very effective, they take a while to kick in. As mentioned previously, you have to wait 4-6 weeks to improve on Tapazole, and 3-4 months on PTU.

Further, your doctor may decide to put you on a dosage of medication that keeps you marginally hyperthyroid. This is often a good strategy if you have one or more goiters, because your TSH has to remain low for the goiters to shrink. But it means you'll still have some remaining symptoms.

Then again, you might be allergic to both Tapazole and PTU. In this case, you'll want some help getting through each day until you're ready for either radioactive iodine treatment or surgery.

In all such situations, you'll require medications to suppress key hyperthyroid problems. Most commonly, you'll need to lower your heart rate. This can be accomplished by a *beta blocker*, which is a drug that blocks the effects of adrenaline, making your heart beat more slowly and with less force. It also helps reduce your blood pressure and improve your blood's circulation. The best beta blockers for hyperthyroidism include *atenolol* and *propranolol*.

You may also be suffering from severe anxiety. This can be managed with anti-anxiety medicines such as *benzodiazepines*, which include Valium, Xanax, Dalmane, and Tranxene. These can be taken regularly several times a day, or only when you feel you need them. However, be aware they can cause drowsiness, affecting how well you drive and decisions you make. Also, they shouldn't be mixed with alcohol or other sedating substances.

Then again, you might do fine on natural remedies that have virtually no side effects, such as magnesium for lowering heart rate, or theanine or kava-kava for calming anxiety.

Block-and-Replace Therapy

If you're on antithyroid medication such as Tapazole, your doctor will monitor you via periodic checkups for 2-3 years until your hyperthyroidism starts petering out on its own. Your doctor will then gradually withdraw your treatment as your thyroid hormone levels lower.

At that point either your thyroid will return to normal, in which case you're home free, or your levels will continue falling, making you hypothyroid. If it becomes clear you're heading in the latter direction, an experienced doctor won't just with-draw treatment and let you plummet into hypothyroidism, but instead will start putting you on low doses of thyroid hormones while you're still being treated for hyperthyroidism.

I call this "driving with the parking brake on," because it allows your doctor to control how quickly you're moving in both directions. It ensures your T4 and T3 levels don't jump up again, while at the same time gently eases you into your new hypothyroid state. It's officially called *block-and-replace therapy*, because your doctor is blocking the disease at the same time that she's replacing any lack of hormones.

After several months or so, your doctor can stop the antithyroid medication entirely, and simply treat you for being hypothyroid. The latter is a cause for celebration, because it essentially means you're out of danger. Once you're hypothyroid, all you have to do is take thyroid medication every morning to maintain healthy hormone levels.

Some doctors are so enthusiastic about block-and-replace therapy that they advocate using it for the entire medication process. Studies don't support this view, though; while it does no harm, this approach doesn't shorten the duration of treatment or improve the outcome. That said, if your T4/T3 levels are continually fluctuating between being too high and too low, block-and-replace therapy is typically the perfect solution.

Radiation and Surgery

Most doctors in Europe greatly prefer using medication to treat hyperthyroidism. In America, however, the first choice of most doctors is *radioiodine ablation*. This uses radioactive iodine to destroy a substantial percentage of the thyroid's cells, making it too small to overproduce hormones.

This works because the thyroid is the only gland in your body that absorbs iodine. When you're given iodine that's radioactive (via pill or injection), the iodine will be ignored by the rest of your body and travel straight to your throat, where it'll be eagerly absorbed by your thyroid cells. The radiation will then kill off the cells.

If your doctor recommends this strategy, he'll probably tell you that there's no risk of developing cancer from it. However, a major study of 2,500 patients followed over 10 years (through 2002) concluded that those who underwent this procedure were later struck by cancer at a 20 percent higher rate than those who didn't. That's a highly significant difference.

Another disadvantage is that your doctor will err on the side of making you hypothyroid. While that's a much safer condition than hyperthyroidism, it's not as good as returning to normal thyroid function; and the latter happens as much as 70 percent of the time for those who choose the medication route.

On the positive side, radioiodine ablation takes 6-18 weeks, while it typically takes 2-3 years of medication and skilled monitoring by your doctor to manage your hyperthyroidism until the disease ends itself naturally.

Further, radioiodine ablation is a tremendously useful option if you're allergic to Tapazole, or if Tapazole simply doesn't happen to work for you. Plus radiation is a straightforward way to reduce the size of goiters, especially if they won't shrink on their own.

I've also found some patients like the apparent finality of radiation over the gradual monitoring and adjustment process of medication. In practice, however, for roughly one out of five patients radioiodine ablation doesn't do the job the first time, requiring a second dose … and increasing the risk of cancer down the line.

In the vast majority of cases, I prefer the medication route for my patients. I find it works with few complications, and it creates no further risk of cancer. But both approaches have positives and negatives.

Finally, you have the option of getting half or all of your thyroid surgically removed. This is considered a last resort, however. While an operation will end your hyperthyroidism, it risks doing damage to your parathyroid glands and vocal chord nerves (see Chapter 13).

Hyperthyroid Patient Stories

It can be easier to understand treatment options when they're viewed within the context of people's lives. The following are true stories of patients who were struggling with hyperthyroidism. They were all restored to full health via medication.

Weary of Radiation

Martha had undergone radioiodine ablation treatment for her Graves' disease … twice. She was still hyperthyroid.

About 20 percent of patients have to return for a second dose of radiation before their T4 and T3 levels fall to normal or hypothyroid levels. But a second treatment not being enough either was pretty unusual. I didn't blame Martha for being frustrated. Further, her doctor was now recommending surgery. Concerned about the risk of complications, she sought me out for a fresh perspective.

Martha was stable on high doses of both Tapazole and the beta blocker atenolol. I told her I'd like to try a slightly different approach for a month and see what happened. After she agreed, I kept Martha on her current medications, but added low doses of fluoride (to block iodine) and lithium (to ease her anxiety). On her first retest, Martha's T4 and T3 levels were in the normal range for the first time in years. She also felt much less anxious.

We moved forward with a medicine-based treatment. Martha continued to improve, and we were able to lower her dosages over the next several months while keeping her T4/T3 levels steady.

Supermeds

Rebecca had a severe case of Graves' disease. Her TSH was <0.01 mIU/L—essentially off the charts—and her free T4 was a sky-high 5.9 ng/dL. I explained that managing her hyperthyroidism would be like stopping a train. It would take the strength of Superman to abruptly bring it to a halt, but after that a simple wheel chock could hold it in place.

I prescribed a high 60 mg daily of Tapazole over the first six weeks to slow down the disease. After that, I was able to bring the dosage down to 10 mg daily for maintenance.

Block and Replace

Peter came to see me for management of his Plummer's disease after unceasing anxiety and panic attacks. His previous doctor had prescribed 20 mg of Tapazole daily, which ended up making Peter hypothyroid. His doctor then prescribed a low dose of Synthroid, which made the hyperthyroidism come back worse than ever.

Afraid of getting even worse, Peter did nothing for six months. Then the misery of his symptoms led him to seek me out for a second opinion. Considering his experiences, I told Peter he'd probably do well on block-and-replace therapy. I prescribed

5 mg of Tapazole and 75 mcg of Synthroid. Within a month, Peter told me he felt like himself again.

Over the following months we made minor adjustments. After Peter had been stable for a full year, I very gradually tapered him off both the Tapazole and Synthroid. He remained healthy. I have Peter keeping a sharp eye out for symptoms, though, and schedule him to see me every six months, just in case there's a recurrence.

The Least You Need to Know

- If your hyperthyroidism is mild, it can be treated with natural remedies such as fluoride, L-carnitine, and goitrogens.

- If your hyperthyroidism symptoms are severe, they can be treated with Tapazole (or its generic version methimazole), or PTU.

- To avoid wild swings toward the end of your hyperthyroidism, your doctor should use block-and-replace therapy.

- If medication isn't effective, you can be treated with radioiodine ablation, which employs radioactive iodine to reduce your thyroid's size; or with surgery.

Other Thyroid Diseases

In this part we provide a step-by-step guide to diagnosing and treating thyroid cancer. The key things to remember are that the most common forms of thyroid cancer have a 97 percent cure rate; and that, as John Diamond wrote, "Cancer is a word, not a sentence."

Chapter 14 covers how to identify and treat problems with your thyroid's partners, the adrenal glands. Chapter 15 tells you about other thyroid-related problems, including parathyroid disease. Chapter 16 describes the devastating emotional effects of thyroid disease, including depression and anxiety. And if you're a woman, Chapter 17 helps you ensure thyroid disease doesn't make a tough time worse when you're experiencing PMS, infertility, postpartum issues, or perimenopause.

Thyroid Cancer

In This Chapter

- Avoiding panic
- Having your thyroid cells examined
- Risks and rewards of surgery
- Understanding your cancer's characteristics
- Obliterating cancer with precision radiation
- Surviving and thriving

One of the scariest words anyone can hear is *cancer*. It's a disease that, like a malicious invader, launches an assault in one area of your body and then keeps expanding its territory, killing everything in its path.

When it comes to thyroid cancer, the good news is that it's rarely fatal. There are around 37,000 cases of thyroid cancer diagnosed in the United States each year, and around 1,600 deaths resulting from it; so the odds for survival are over 95 percent. That's because the most common forms of thyroid cancer grow slowly, and so can usually be stopped via surgical removal of one or both of your thyroid's lobes before the cancer spreads to other parts of your body. If only one of your lobes needs to be removed, the other will probably be able to take on the work of producing your thyroid hormones by itself. Alternatively, if the entire thyroid has to be removed, your doctors can usually exploit the unique characteristics of thyroid cells to target any remnants of the cancer post-surgery and destroy them.

One of the most challenging aspects of thyroid cancer is dealing with the fear and stress it brings. This chapter will help you understand the process for evaluation and treatment, empowering you to ask the right questions and make the best decisions ... and giving you the peace of mind of knowing that the odds are enormously in your favor.

THROAT QUOTE

Cancer is a word, not a sentence.

—John Diamond

Noticing Nodules

There's a saying among doctors: "If it hurts, it's probably not cancer." You can have thyroid cancer and not know it for years, because you're unlikely to feel it or have it substantially affect your thyroid's ability to function. In fact, it's not unusual for someone to die of unrelated causes and be discovered to have thyroid cancer only upon postmortem examination.

The primary sign of thyroid cancer is one or more masses, called *nodules*, growing on the thyroid. They're typically noticed when one of them grows big enough to be seen or felt through the throat. A nodule might also call attention to itself by growing large enough to give you trouble swallowing, or by pressing on your vocal nerves to make your voice hoarse.

By age 50, roughly 50 percent of us have one or more thyroid nodules; and over 95 percent of the time, these nodules are harmless. But when a nodule grows large enough to be noticed, it's important to have a doctor check it out for safety's sake. This is because while thyroid cancer cells typically duplicate themselves slowly, each duplication doubles the size of the mass. It can take decades for a few pioneering cancer cells to duplicate enough times to become a significant nodule; but at that point, even though the rate of duplication remains the same, the doubling effect means the cancer cells have to be dealt with because they might soon spread beyond your thyroid.

So even though the odds are against a nodule being cancerous, the possibility shouldn't be ignored. That's especially the case if you're a woman, as you're three times as likely to develop thyroid cancer as a man, and if you're age 30 or over, as both the risk of having thyroid cancer and its severity increase as you get older.

Taking an Initial Look

There's nothing you can do on your own to evaluate a nodule, so you need to see a doctor. You can start with your general practitioner, or go straight to a specialist—which in this case is an ear, nose, and throat (ENT) surgeon.

Either way, your doctor will typically perform a manual exam, take some blood to send to a lab for thyroid testing, and then prescribe an ultrasound test. You shouldn't hesitate to agree to the latter, as it's relatively quick and inexpensive—and it doesn't involve radiation, so it's entirely safe.

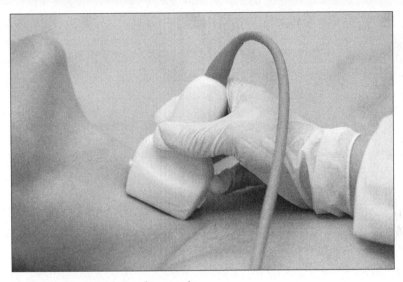

Checking the thyroid via ultrasound.
(Licensed from Shutterstock Images)

An ultrasound lets your doctor see what's going on inside your throat by bouncing high-frequency sound waves off your thyroid (similar to how bats and submarines use sound to navigate). A technician will lubricate your throat with jelly to make the sound waves transmit more effectively, and then move a handheld component of the machine over your throat to take pictures of your thyroid, including its nodules.

A specialist will then examine the images, looking for such details as whether a nodule is entirely filled with fluid (in which case it might be a mere cyst), or if it's one of a number of nodules the same size (which could mean you have a benign multi-nodule goiter), or whether it's solid and attached to an unusually large number of veins (which is cause for suspicion as cancer is greedy for blood, making new blood vessels form just to feed itself).

Alternatively, if your doctor suspects you're hyperthyroid, he may prescribe an iodine uptake and thyroid scan, which involves taking a tiny amount of radioactive iodine. The radiation will "light up" whatever absorbs it, and the only things in your body that absorb iodine are thyroid cells. If a nodule is causing your hyperthyroidism, it'll show up as "hot," meaning it absorbed the iodine and is probably responsible for your having too many thyroid hormones. If a nodule is "cold," however—meaning it's not absorbing the iodine and making no hormones—that's cause for suspicion, as some types of cancer cells don't use iodine and produce nothing except more cancer cells. About 10 percent of "cold" nodules turn out to be cancerous.

If your ultrasound or uptake scan provides enough information to consider your nodule(s) benign, then you can stop exploring the possibility of cancer for now. However, you should see your doctor at least once a year so she can monitor your thyroid and note whether there's any further growth.

On the other hand, if the testing leaves room for suspicion, this is the time to start looking for an ENT surgeon who has long experience and a great reputation for diagnosing and, if necessary, dealing with thyroid cancer.

Getting a Biopsy

The next step in checking your nodule(s) is a *fine needle aspiration biopsy.* This involves your ENT doctor taking a very thin—and relatively painless—needle attached to a syringe and sticking it into your throat, aiming for every major nodule on your thyroid (usually based on his feeling its location, or sometimes with the aid of an ultrasound machine).

For each insertion, you'll be asked to hold your breath so your doctor can gently rock the needle back and forth to gather as much tissue as possible. Your doctor will then retract the syringe to capture small bits of tissue from the nodule. He'll repeat this procedure 2-6 times for each large nodule. This is a quick procedure that's usually performed in your doctor's office, and when done properly isn't much more of a bother than getting an injection.

The samples from your biopsy will be sent to a *cytopathologist,* who's an expert at evaluating minute clues about cells. The cytopathologist will carefully examine your samples under a microscope, and will then reach one of four conclusions:

- You don't have thyroid cancer and your nodule's cells show no signs of cancer. This happens about 70 percent of the time.

- You do have thyroid cancer and your doctor's needle captured cells that are clearly cancerous. This happens about 5-10 percent of the time.

- Not enough thyroid tissue was gathered to make an analysis. This happens about 10 percent of the time.

- No cells were found that are definitively cancerous, but there are cells with suspicious characteristics. This happens about 10-15 percent of the time.

The first three situations are relatively straightforward. If the cytopathologist finds no significant signs of cancer, the chances are over 95 percent that you're fine. Simply be sure to visit your general practitioner every six months to check on whether there's been any nodule growth.

Alternatively, if the cytopathologist determines you have cancer, the chances she's right are also over 95 percent (and if she's highly experienced, closer to 100 percent). This isn't a cause for panic, as most thyroid cancer is as treatable as cancer gets; but it does mean you'll need surgery. (More on this shortly.)

If not enough useable tissue was gathered, then the biopsy has to be repeated. This isn't unheard of. However, you might want to have a discussion with your ENT about what went wrong; and at the same time casually ask how many thyroid biopsies he's performed. If your doctor hasn't already handled hundreds of thyroid cancer cases, consider finding one who has.

The most complicated situation is when the cytopathologist has enough tissue to work with, but still can't make a definitive judgment. This can happen for a number of reasons. For example, you might have thyroid cancer, but your doctor didn't happen to capture cancer cells during any of his needle insertions (a nodule can contain both cancerous and benign cells). However, he captured nearby cells that hint at the presence of cancer. Or your sample might consist of follicular cells. Follicular cancer comprises around 12 percent of all thyroid cancers, but a biopsy is incapable of providing enough information to distinguish between cancerous and noncancerous follicular cells.

When faced with this gray area, the only way to find out for certain whether a nodule is cancerous is to surgically remove it and place it under a microscope. However, the surgery carries significant risks (described below). And in over 75 percent of these cases, the nodule turns out to be benign.

At the same time, there's also a risk in letting a nodule that might be cancerous continue to grow … and potentially spread beyond your thyroid. This is a situation in which you want a deeply experienced ENT doctor to advise you. You should ask for a copy of the cytopathologist's report and have your doctor explain the details behind the finding of "indeterminate."

THYROIDIAN TIP

Another pre-surgery test worth asking about is a *coarse needle biopsy,* which allows for the removal of a greater amount of thyroid tissue than fine needle aspiration for nodules three quarters of an inch or larger. Not all doctors are qualified to perform this procedure; but when used as a follow-up for certain types of indeterminate results, coarse needle biopsies have been found to significantly reduce unnecessary thyroid surgeries.

You might also want to get a second opinion. Surgery on your throat isn't something to take lightly, and neither is cancer; so don't hesitate to gather more information before making a decision.

Selecting Surgery

If your biopsy showed you have thyroid cancer, or if the results were sufficiently suspicious to justify pursuing a definitive answer, your next step is to have surgery.

If you choose this route, you'll first be placed under anesthesia. Your ENT surgeon will then open your neck and *very* carefully work on your thyroid. This is a delicate procedure because there are some critical body parts nearby. Specifically, the nerves for your vocal chords are right next to your thyroid. If these nerves are pulled too hard or otherwise injured, it will impair your ability to speak. The results can be a hoarse or whispery voice, with reduced power and/or range. In most cases the condition is temporary, but there are rare instances when the damage is permanent. This is a major reason to choose an ENT who has performed many previous thyroid surgeries.

Also at risk are your *parathyroids,* which are small glands residing behind your thyroid that regulate the amount of calcium in your blood and bones (see Chapter 15). The precise location, number, and size of these glands varies from person to person, increasing the odds of accidentally damaging one or more of them. Thyroid surgeons focus heavily on protecting the parathyroids, so the likelihood of permanent harm is small, but temporary injury is a real possibility, happening to around 8 percent of patients. (A telltale sign is tingling or numbness in your fingers, toes, or lips within the first few days following surgery.) Even if you feel no symptoms, you'll be told to take calcium supplements for a month following the surgery to lighten the strain on your parathyroids in case they need time to recover.

During surgery, your doctor first explores your thyroid to spot all nodules and anything else suspicious. If this inspection makes it apparent that you have cancer on both lobes, then he'll remove the entire thyroid.

Otherwise, first the lobe with the largest (or only) nodule is removed. If you're in a top facility with both a cytopathologist and cytology lab available for the operation—which is ideal—the lobe's cells are examined while you're still under anesthesia, providing your surgeon with definitive information about whether there's cancer present and, if so, what type of cancer. Your surgeon can then decide whether to remove the rest of your thyroid or to allow the second lobe to remain. In the latter case you'll probably still have a fully functioning thyroid (with the remaining lobe simply doing twice the amount of the work as before).

If your hospital doesn't have the resources to check your thyroid's cells during the operation, though, then your doctor may remove one lobe, end the operation, and wait until a cytopathologist examines the lobe to decide if you need a second operation to take out the rest of your thyroid.

Alternatively, if the results of your biopsy strongly indicate cancer, you and your doctor may decide pre-surgery that he'll remove the entire thyroid. This spares you from undergoing a second operation and provides peace of mind that the cancer won't spread—but at the cost of a functioning thyroid that might never become cancerous. The pros and cons of this decision vary depending on such factors as the type of cancer involved (some are more aggressive than others) and your age (thyroid cancer becomes more dangerous as you get older).

Types of Thyroid Cancer

After you've had surgery, sections of your removed nodule(s) will be studied by a cytopathologist to determine precisely what sort of thyroid cancer caused them. This is important information because it'll help determine what additional steps need to be taken.

The primary possibilities are no cancer, papillary, follicular, and medullary. (There are other types, but they collectively account for less than 5 percent of thyroid cancer cases.)

No Cancer

After removing half your thyroid, your doctor may find the nodule(s) growing on it to be benign. As mentioned previously, this happens over 75 percent of the time. You may feel bad about losing a healthy thyroid lobe, as well as risking your vocal chords and parathyroids; but you may also feel glad about having the peace of mind of knowing you're cancer-free.

Either way, you still have half of a functioning thyroid, and there's a good chance it'll make all the thyroid hormone you need. For safety's sake, however, keep a lookout for hypothyroid symptoms (see Chapter 6). Also take care to get your thyroid hormone levels tested after six months, and then annually, in case you eventually become hypothyroid as a result of your remaining lobe doing twice as much work as it was designed for.

Papillary Cancer

Papillary is by far the most common form of thyroid cancer, accounting for about 80 percent of cases. It typically stems from exposure to radiation. It's slow growing, taking 10-20 years to develop to the point where it's noticeable.

It's also *well differentiated*, meaning it closely resembles normal thyroid cells. For example, papillary cancer absorbs iodine like a normal thyroid cell—which means it's ideally suited for destruction by radioactive iodine (see the next section, "Getting Radioactive").

Papillary cancer tends to stay in the neck—for instance, invading the lymph nodes. However, around 5-10 percent of patients eventually develop papillary cancer in other areas of their body, particularly the lungs and bones. So even though it's slow growing, this cancer has to be taken seriously and destroyed before it spreads.

Follicular Cancer

Follicular is the second most common form of thyroid cancer, accounting for around 12 percent of cases. Its causes are believed to include radiation, genetics, and low iodine consumption.

Like papillary, follicular cancer is well differentiated, absorbing iodine like normal thyroid cells—which means it's also ideally suited for destruction by radioactive iodine.

Follicular cancer doesn't tend to spread in the neck, but around 20 percent of patients eventually develop it in the lungs and bones.

Medullary Cancer

Medullary is the third most common form of thyroid cancer, accounting for around 5 percent of cases. Its causes are unknown beyond genetics; about 25 percent of people struck by it have a family history of the disease.

Medullary cancer is *not* well differentiated, so it doesn't absorb iodine like a normal thyroid cell and won't be affected by radioactive iodine. It's also not affected by chemotherapy.

Medullary cancer is substantially more aggressive than papillary and follicular, invading lymph nodes over 50 percent of the time.

The best method for eliminating medullary cancer is surgery—removing the entire thyroid, possibly the lymph nodes, and anywhere else it appears to have invaded. Follow-up visits to check for any recurrence is mandatory. If the cancer comes back, the best option is usually more surgery. However, sometimes radiation can also be effective.

Getting Radioactive

One of the advantages of getting your entire thyroid removed is it makes you a candidate for *radioactive iodine treatment*. This is a clever way to destroy papillary and follicular cancer (making up about 92 percent of thyroid cancer cases) by taking advantage of one of the unique properties of the thyroid.

Specifically, the thyroid is the only gland in your body that absorbs iodine. And although your thyroid was removed, many of its cells are still in your throat … including cancerous ones. To deal with this, after surgery you won't be allowed thyroid medication for 4-6 weeks. This will put you into a severe hypothyroid state—and make your thyroid cells starved for iodine.

You'll then be given a single dose of radioactive iodine (usually via a small pill encased in an impressively large and heavy lead container). Although the pill looks ordinary, it's so radioactive that you'll be told to avoid living things—people and pets—for 48 hours after taking it. You'll also be told to suck on sour candies, which will prevent the radiation from doing damage to your salivary glands. (Don't spit on anything, though, as your saliva—and, for that matter, your clothes—will be radioactive for the next 30 days.)

The iodine from the pill will be ignored by the rest of your body and travel straight to your throat, where it'll be eagerly absorbed by whatever thyroid cells remain. If you have papillary or follicular cancer, its cells absorb the iodine … and the radiation will obliterate them. (It'll also kill whatever benign thyroid cells remain; but since your thyroid is now gone, that doesn't matter.)

THYROIDIAN TIP

Thyroid cancer cells will typically be confined to your throat. If they've spread to other parts of your body, though, they'll attract and absorb their share of the radioactive iodine and it'll annihilate them as well.

If all goes well, this treatment will make you cancer-free, eliminating the possibility of stray thyroid cancer cells eventually spreading to other parts of your body. The only downside is the same as that carried by any radiation treatment—long-term, it poses the risk of initiating cancer itself. But in this case, the positive outcome of annihilating cancer that exists here and now more than makes up for the remote possibility of developing cancer years later from the radiation.

Treatment for Life

If your entire thyroid is removed, you've effectively become hypothyroid. You'll therefore need to take thyroid medication—typically, a pill or two every morning—for the rest of your life.

You can find information about medication options in Chapters 8 and 9. In your case, your first choice should be desiccated thyroid, or a mix of desiccated and synthetic thyroid. Synthetic medications (e.g., Synthroid and Cytomel) can be fine if your thyroid is still partially functioning, but since it's not, desiccated thyroid is the only way for your body to obtain not only T4 and T3, but also a normal amount of T2 (which has been found to be significant for metabolism and weight loss) and T1 (which so far has no known use, but is being studied).

You should also make a point of seeing your doctor every 6-12 months for follow-up visits. That's especially true if you've had radioactive iodine therapy, as there's a special test you can take a year following the treatment to check on whether it's been successful. Meanwhile, feel comforted in knowing the chances are around 97 percent that it has, and that you're entirely healthy again.

Julie's Story

If you'd like a down-to-earth example of what going through the diagnostic and treatment process is like, the experience of my patient Julie is fairly typical.

While curling her hair shortly after her 38th birthday, Julie noticed a lump the size of a marble protruding from her neck. She thought it was quite prominent and was surprised she hadn't spotted it before. Then it occurred to Julie that it might have grown quickly. She realized it could be serious and needed to be checked out.

Julie's family doctor saw her the following week. After feeling her throat, he told her it was probably just a swollen lymph node. "These things happen all the time," he said. "Don't worry about it; but come back next month if it's still there."

A week later Julie's lump had clearly grown larger, so she made another appointment with her doctor. When he examined her neck again, he found the lump was now over 1 centimeter. "I'm sending you to get an ultrasound," he said. "That'll help us know what's going on."

The ultrasound was arranged for the following week. While waiting for it, Julie could think of little else. During her test Julie tried to get some information from the face of the technician, but he was unreadable. After it was done she asked him what he thought. "All I can do is take the images," he said. "I'm not qualified to evaluate. But your doctor will receive the results within a few days."

In fact, Julie's doctor called her the next day. "It's not a lymph node," he said. "It's a thyroid nodule. I'm referring you to an ENT."

The next week Julie was seen by an ear, nose, and throat surgeon. After a manual exam, he conducted a fine needle aspiration biopsy, taking six tiny samples of Julie's nodule with a needle and syringe. Although Julie pressed, the doctor was unwilling to make any guesses about her condition. "I'll probably have the results tomorrow, though," he said. "I'll call you when they come in."

The next day Julie was unable to concentrate on anything as she waited anxiously for the call. She hoped it would happen in the morning, but it didn't. She stayed by her desk during lunch, just in case. When 4 P.M. rolled by, Julie stopped waiting and called the doctor's office. "I'm glad you got in touch," the receptionist said. "The doctor had tried to call you, but it looks like two digits of your phone number accidentally got transposed. Let me put you through now." After a moment, Julie was on the line with the ENT.

Julie first thought from his calm tone of voice that the results came back negative. Then he told her, "You tested positive for papillary cancer of the thyroid. However, the cells don't appear to be very aggressive." All Julie really heard at that moment was "You have cancer."

The following day Julie met with the ENT, and he calmly assured her that her odds were excellent. "The surgery alone will probably cure you," he said. "But we'll give you a dose of radiation afterward to be extra safe. With your permission, I'll make the arrangements."

Given the schedule of the ENT and the anesthesiologist, plus Julie needing prior authorization from her insurance provider, the operation was scheduled to take place in three weeks. Julie began to feel everyone was taking this far too casually. During the three weeks she did little other than fixate on the lump of foreign poison she felt was going to end her life.

When the ENT performed the surgery, he found two nodules—the one that had already been noticed, which had since grown to over 2 centimeters, and another one that was 1.5 centimeters. They were both on the left lobe;, but based on a discussion with Julie before the operation, the ENT removed her entire thyroid so Julie could feel certain the cancer wouldn't spread.

When Julie woke up afterward, the ENT told her the operation was a success. He also told her that she wouldn't be given thyroid hormones for six weeks "so when you take the radioactive iodine, any remaining cancer cells will suck it up like a vacuum cleaner."

Six weeks later, in a hypothyroid state that had made her thoroughly fatigued and 10 pounds heavier, Julie was given 130 millicuries of radioactive iodine. She stayed away from people and other living things for two days. During this time there was some swelling under her jaw, but sucking on sour candies made it go away.

Afterward Julie made an appointment with an endocrinologist and was overjoyed to finally be allowed to take thyroid medication.

Over the next couple of months Julie was relieved that the surgery, the radiation, and most importantly the cancer were behind her. However, she noticed clear continuing symptoms of fatigue; plus her hair started thinning, and she was starting to feel inexplicably depressed. Her endocrinologist told her that according to the blood tests her thyroid dosage was fine, so nothing else needed to be done.

After a few more months, Julie's hair started falling out. No longer trusting her endocrinologist, Julie sought me out. I found she was actually still hypothyroid due to her medication dosage being too low, and also being exclusively T4 (i.e., with no T3 or T2).

I switched Julie to desiccated thyroid and a higher dosage. Within two months Julie felt entirely healthy again.

The Least You Need to Know

- Thyroid cancer is about as treatable as cancer gets, with a survival rate of over 95 percent.

- Ultrasound and fine needle aspiration biopsy are the best ways to explore a thyroid nodule.

- If you need surgery, get the most experienced ear, nose, and throat (ENT) surgeon you can find.

- If you have your entire thyroid removed, don't hesitate to obliterate remaining cancer cells with radioactive cancer treatment.

- For the two most common types of thyroid cancer, papillary and follicular, the cure rate is 97 percent.

- If your entire thyroid is removed, choose desiccated thyroid medication to fully replace its hormones (T4, T3, T2, and T1).

Adrenal Gland Diseases

In This Chapter

- Understanding the thyroid-adrenal connection
- Recognizing adrenal disease symptoms
- Best testing strategies
- Healing underperforming adrenals
- Dealing with overperforming adrenals

As explained in Chapter 7, it's possible to be hypothyroid but labeled "normal" on blood tests because the ranges used by most labs are too broad. To make life even more complicated, you can be hypothyroid and labeled "normal" on blood tests because your thyroid really *is* functioning normally. This paradox stems from a pair of endocrine glands called adrenals that your thyroid relies on to be effective.

Spotlighting Your Adrenal Glands

The adrenal glands are two small triangle-shaped lumps of tissue residing over your kidneys.

The adrenal glands are divided into four sections: an outer *cortex* with three layers, and an inner *medulla*. Each section produces hormones regulating bodily functions vital to your health. These can be summarized as *salt*, *sugar*, *sex*, and *stress*:

- **Salt:** The outermost cortex layer produces hormones such as *aldosterone* that control the amount of sodium and water in your body, and regulate your blood pressure.

- **Sugar:** The middle cortex layer makes the critical hormone *cortisol*, whose many functions include regulating your blood's glucose levels (along with your pancreas), controlling your blood pressure (along with aldosterone), healing inflammations, and enabling your thyroid hormones to enter cells.

- **Sex:** The innermost cortex layer creates the sex hormones testosterone and estrogen (as a backup for your testicles or ovaries, which produce the same sex hormones).

- **Stress:** The medulla produces *adrenaline*, a hormone that's triggered when you're in a dangerous or unexpected situation. Adrenaline increases your heart rate, expands your blood vessels and air passages, and makes other subtle changes that help you react instantly to whatever trouble comes your way by either battling or running (commonly called *fight or flight*).

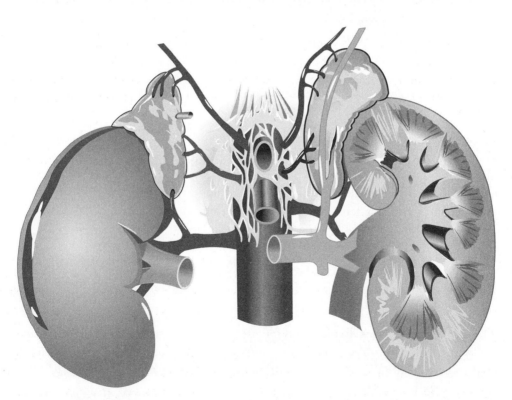

The adrenal glands.
(Licensed from Shutterstock Images)

When a Good Thyroid Seems Bad

The adrenal hormone most important to your thyroid is cortisol, which plays two vital roles. First, cortisol helps convert the T4 that leaves your thyroid (or that you're taking via medication) into T3. That's a vital function, because T4 is merely a storage state; your body can only make use of T3. In addition, cortisol gives T3 the ability to penetrate a cell's membrane. Once inside a cell, the T3 powers up the cell's mitochondria, providing your body with the energy it needs.

The partnership between your thyroid and your adrenals works beautifully when both glands are healthy. If your adrenal glands start underperforming, however, there won't be enough cortisol to convert T4 into all the T3 you need. Worse, there won't be enough cortisol to allow T3 to penetrate your cells. That means even if your thyroid is doing its job perfectly, your body won't benefit from it because a certain amount of T3 will be blocked from accessing your mitochondria.

Conversely, if your adrenal glands are overperforming, then you'll have too much cortisol in your system, and that's just as much of a problem, because excessive cortisol prevents mitochondria from absorbing thyroid hormones. The result is the same—the mitochondria don't get recharged, depriving you of energy vital to your health.

In either case, you'll end up in a hypothyroid state. Your thyroid blood tests will all show up as normal—because your thyroid really *is* healthy and performing its job perfectly. What needs to be diagnosed and treated are your adrenal glands.

Underactive Adrenals

If your adrenal glands are underperforming, you may have *Addison's disease* (also called *adrenal insufficiency*). This refers to a physical problem with your adrenals, such as a genetic defect, or an autoimmune disorder in which your adrenals are being attacked by antibodies. Addison's disease is relatively rare, affecting 1 to 4 out of every 100,000 people.

Alternatively, you might have a problem with your pituitary gland, which controls the activity of your adrenals via a hormone called *ACTH* (also known as *adrenocorticotropic hormone* or *corticotropin*). If for some reason your pituitary starts producing too little ACTH, your adrenal glands—even though perfectly healthy—will underperform because they're following the "orders" conveyed by the ACTH. This is called *secondary adrenal insufficiency*, as the cause is indirect—it's really your pituitary that has the problem, but your adrenals behave as if they're ailing. Further, if this condition is left untreated, over time your adrenals really *will* become damaged, as they'll shrink from lack of use. This condition is much more common than Addison's disease.

Another cause for underperformance is a shortage of the chemical building blocks that fuel hormone production. For example, your adrenals require cholesterol to make cortisol. If your body is having trouble getting cholesterol to your adrenals, or if you're taking medication that interferes with cholesterol, your adrenal glands won't have enough raw material to do their job.

As another example of underperformance, your adrenal glands are secondary suppliers of the sex hormones testosterone and estrogen, essentially backing up the primary production from your testicles or ovaries. At the age when women begin menopause and men's testicles start producing less testosterone (sometimes referred to as *andro-pause*), the adrenals are required to pick up the slack. If there was a barely adequate amount of chemical ingredients to work with to start, the increased demand for sex hormones will force the adrenals to cut back on other hormones—including cortisol. For this reason, if you're going to have an adrenal problem, it's most likely to happen around age 45-55.

Finally, some doctors believe the number one source of adrenal problems is *adrenal fatigue*, or *hypoadrenalism*, which occurs as a three-stage process. When life hands you the occasional hardship, your adrenals will produce extra hormones to help you get through it and will then return to normal. This first stage is called *compensation*, and is perfectly healthy. If such strains become frequent, though, or if they become exceptionally severe, your adrenals are likely to overreact and produce more hormones than are good for you. This stage is called *overcompensation*. If the stress then continues over a long period of time, the wear and tear on your adrenals may eventually cause them to lose the ability to produce even normal levels of hormones. This third stage is called *decompensation*.

If this happens to you, your adrenals are likely to *subtly* underperform—not create symptoms as severe as those of Addison's disease, but still impair your quality of life. The good news is adrenal fatigue can often be managed with over-the-counter remedies that have virtually no side effects.

Identifying Underactivity

Because your adrenal glands regulate blood sugar, salt, blood pressure, and stress responses, there are some quick and easy things you can do on your own as a first rough check on whether they're underperforming.

First, try delaying or skipping a meal and see if it's any harder to do than usual. If so, that could mean you've become *hypoglycemic*—low on blood sugar—which in turn could mean a shortage of cortisol. Also notice if you have any other symptoms of hypoglycemia, which include frequent hunger (especially for sugar or starch), fatigue, impaired judgment, confusion, nausea, anxiety, and shakiness. In addition, note whether you've developed strong cravings for salt. That can indicate a shortage of the adrenal hormone aldosterone.

Next, perform a quick check on your blood pressure. It's easy to take your body's management of blood pressure for granted; but when you stand up, there's actually quite a bit of complex internal orchestration involved to prevent your blood from abruptly dropping from your brain into your feet. When the adrenal hormones cortisol and aldosterone are low, this mechanism isn't as effective; so try lying down for a few minutes and then abruptly rising. If you become dizzy, feel weak, and/or see spots, it's probably because more blood rushed down from your brain than is normal.

THYROIDIAN TIP

If you'd prefer a more formal version of the blood pressure test, tell your doctor that you want her to check your *orthostatic hypotension*. She'll have you lie down, hook you up to a blood pressure machine, and then ask you to stand. If you're healthy, your systolic (top number) blood pressure will go up 5-10 points. But if you're low on adrenal hormones, it'll drop 10-25 points.

Another test you can perform easily on your own is checking your fight-or-flight response, which is regulated by the hormone adrenaline. First sit in front of a mirror and turn off the light for a minute, which will make your pupils open wide. Then shine a flashlight across (but not directly into) your eyes, and watch how your pupils react for the next 30 seconds. Your irises should instantly contract in response to the light increasing, and stay contracted. If you're low on adrenaline, however, it's likely that your irises will contract briefly but then expand; or waver back and forth between contracting and expanding.

One other way you can identify underperforming adrenals is paying attention to your skin (and especially your torso's epidermis). A combination of low cortisol and high ACTH can stimulate the cells that control skin pigmentation, resulting in dark, irregularly shaped spots a few inches long—sometimes called "café au lait spots" because they look like spilled coffee.

Testing for Underactivity

If you have reason to suspect an adrenal problem, you should visit an endocrinologist for formal testing. Your doctor will test your cortisol levels. Unfortunately, this isn't a straightforward procedure, because cortisol varies over the course of a day. If you're on a mainstream schedule, your cortisol level will rise in the morning, peaking at around 7 A.M., and then sink to very low levels at night. Your doctor will therefore probably take two blood tests—one in the morning and the other in the afternoon—noting the time of day for each so that can be factored in when evaluating the lab results.

If you happen to work at night and sleep during the day, however, your cortisol patterns might be reversed. And if your schedule shifts from day to day, that makes taking just a couple of blood tests even more problematic. To get around this, some doctors will ask you to collect your urine over a 24-hour period. The total is then tested to determine the cortisol level *on average* for the entire day. The downside is there's no information on highs and lows—that is, how much the cortisol varied from one time of day to another. Therefore, this test is most useful as a supplement to the twice-a-day blood test.

Another approach is what's called a *cortisol challenge test*. This involves measuring your cortisol level; giving you a small (typically 25 microgram) dose of ACTH, which is the hormone your pituitary gland makes to stimulate adrenal activity; waiting an hour or two; and then measuring your cortisol level again. If your adrenal glands are healthy, they should have produced at least twice as much cortisol in response to the ACTH. If they didn't, it's a strong indicator they're ailing. This is an excellent way of obtaining precise information about adrenal performance.

This technique is also useful if you have physical symptoms of adrenal underperformance but your cortisol levels don't appear significantly off-kilter on standard blood tests. Even if you have a tolerable cortisol level when you're sitting calmly in a doctor's office, the challenge test will show if your adrenals are inadequate when faced with stress or other demanding situations that call for extra hormone production.

One other available option is *salivary cortisol testing*. This allows you to enjoy a normal day, but take a sample of your saliva every 4-6 hours (using a kit supplied by your doctor), marking the time each sample is taken. Adrenal hormones in your saliva are roughly proportional to those in your blood, so the test results allow your doctor to track your cortisol levels throughout the day. The main disadvantage of this method is hormones attach to red blood cells. It's common to have tiny amounts of blood in the saliva, and even if they're too small to see, they can skew results. But your doctor can instruct you on ways to minimize this problem (such as not brushing your teeth the day of the testing).

> **THYROIDIAN TIP**
>
> It's possible to be hypothyroid from thyroid disease alone and from adrenal disease alone. But you shouldn't discount the possibility of having *both* diseases. If your thyroid starts failing, your adrenals may work harder in an attempt to compensate and eventually become damaged from the strain. So if you notice symptoms of both diseases, it might not be your imagination, and you shouldn't hesitate to get tested for both.

Treating Underactivity

The standard treatment for low cortisol levels is cortisol replacement medication. However, this isn't an ideal solution. Your body needs different amounts of cortisol at different hours of the day. In addition, it requires extra cortisol when you're faced with challenging situations, such as stress or an infection. Taking a pill once a day is a poor substitute for the flexibility and adaptability provided by your adrenal glands.

Further, consuming external cortisol can create new health problems. Cortisol is an anti-inflammatory, so it will stop inflammation wherever it ends up in your body. Since inflammation is an important tool your body uses to repair itself, prolonged use of cortisol replacement risks erosion of your intestinal lining and esophagus.

If your adrenal glands are severely damaged—for example, if you have advanced Addison's disease—then taking cortisol pills for life may be your only realistic option. If you have a choice, though, it's better to first try making your adrenals stronger and more efficient.

For example, taking the herb *ashwagandha* (Latin name *withania somnifera*) poses virtually no risk of side effects; and it increases the odds of your adrenal glands restoring themselves to normal over time. (Plus if you have other glands that are ailing—including your thyroid—ashwagandha is likely to help them, too.)

Another simple but helpful aid is licorice, which is powerfully effective at delaying the conversion of cortisol to cortisone. This helps you hang on to the cortisol your body is making on its own.

Yet another potential solution is taking adrenal tissue—typically from cows—in tablet form. Some studies have found that if you orally ingest a gland, your body will make use of it to shore up your own version of the gland.

Finally, you can make lifestyle changes that ease the strain on your adrenals, such as eating healthy, cutting down on stress, and eliminating toxins. For details, see Chapters 18 and 22.

Overactive Adrenals

As bad as it is to have too little cortisol, it's even worse to have too much of it. The latter condition is called *Cushing's syndrome*, or *hypercortisolism*. Cushing's syndrome often results from cortisol-based medication such as prednisone. Because of its anti-inflammatory properties, cortisol is used to treat such illnesses as asthma, rheumatoid arthritis, lupus, and ulcerative colitis. That's normally fine; but if you take high doses of cortisol for a prolonged period, it will start to break down your tissues, and may do damage to your heart and bones. If this occurs, you can simply taper off your current medication and then switch to one that's not cortisol-based.

More serious is when your adrenal glands are overproducing cortisol. This is relatively rare, occurring most often in adults aged 20-50. It also happens in women in the last trimester of pregnancy, as that's a period of substantial hormone changes. Causes include autoimmune disease, in which antibodies attack your adrenals and cause them to enlarge.

Alternatively, your adrenal glands' cells can spawn tumors called *pheochromocytoma*—growing either on the glands or outside of them—that produce hormones independently. The combination of hormones from both your adrenals and the tumors will put you beyond healthy limits.

A more indirect cause that ends up creating the same effect is your body having too much ACTH. This can happen if you're taking medication that contains a high amount of ACTH. It can also result from *adenomas* (non-cancerous tumors) that start growing on your pituitary gland and increase ACTH output. In either case, the extra ACTH forces your adrenals to produce more cortisol than is good for you.

CRASH GLANDING

The pituitary gland isn't the only source of ACTH. Extra ACTH can also stem from cancerous tumors—for example, in the lungs or intestines. When this occurs, the symptoms of Cushing's syndrome are actually a blessing, because they'll tip off an astute doctor to the existence of cancers that must be located and destroyed.

Alternatively, you can lead your adrenals to develop bad habits. For example, if you're an athlete who trains hard, you're forcing your adrenal glands to produce a lot of extra cortisol. That's usually not a problem if you take care to include adequate periods in between sessions for your body to rest, recover, and reset. But if you're overtraining day after day, your adrenal glands can become so used to overgenerating cortisol that they get stuck at that higher setting and will continue to overproduce even if you stop exercising.

Identifying Overactivity

The primary symptom of Cushing's syndrome is gaining a lot of weight, especially in the middle and upper body. Fat is prone to gather around the neck and back (between the shoulder blades). In children, the obesity is accompanied by a slowed rate of growth. In addition, there's often facial swelling that creates a rounded "moon face." At the same time, loss of lean body mass results in relatively thin arms and legs.

Further, too much cortisol thins the skin, making it easy for mere bumps to bruise or tear skin. The fragility of the skin, coupled with the weight gain, can also result in pink or purple stretch marks on the torso, arms, buttocks, thighs, legs, and/or breasts. Thinning, brittle hair and hair loss is common as well.

Because cortisol reduces immune responses, wounds may happen more often and take an extra long time to heal. You could also start developing aches and pains in your hips, shoulders, and lower back. And you might be the first to catch any illness going around and among the last to recover.

Your adrenals producing excess adrenaline can heighten and intensify your emotions, making you feel anxious, euphoric, depressed, or even psychotic.

If you're a woman, your adrenals overproducing sex hormones can cause your menstrual cycles to become irregular, or to stop altogether. Further, you might get unusual patterns of hair growth and facial acne. And if you're a man, the overdose of cortisol can reduce your sex drive and impair erections.

Additional symptoms include high blood sugar, increased thirst and urination, fatigue, weakness, and hypertension.

Cushing's syndrome must be taken seriously. If left untreated for a long time, it can lead to diabetes, osteoporosis, heart disease, and death.

Testing for Overactivity

Your doctor will typically check for adrenal overproduction by giving you 1 milligram of dexamethasone, which is a powerful synthetic version of cortisol, and then testing your blood's cortisol levels both the same day and the next day. If you're healthy, your pituitary gland should pick up on the fact your body has more cortisol than it needs and lower its production of ACTH. If your blood test the following day doesn't show reduced cortisol, then your pituitary gland has a problem, some other part of your body (typically, a tumor) is generating ACTH on its own, or your adrenals aren't responding normally to the ACTH.

Other ways to test your cortisol levels are to have you collect either your urine or your saliva over a 24-hour period. If your doctor determines there's a problem, she'll order a CT scan of your adrenals and MRI of your pituitary gland to hone in on it, looking for anything out of the ordinary such as growths on the glands.

Treating Overactivity

There are some drugs that either lower the body's production of cortisol or lower the effects of cortisol, such as ketoconazole and metyrapone. However, their effectiveness is limited.

Therefore, the most common solution is surgery. For example, if an adenoma is found on the pituitary gland, the growth will be cut out. If the surgery restores your glands to health, then nothing more needs to be done.

However, if the surgery either removed or damaged your pituitary or adrenal glands, you'll need to deal with a shortage of cortisol (as described earlier in this chapter).

The Least You Need to Know

- If you have clear hypothyroid symptoms but your thyroid tests are normal, you may have adrenal gland disease.
- Symptoms of underperforming adrenals include low blood sugar, salt cravings, dizziness when abruptly standing up, and coffee-stain-like spots on your skin.
- Symptoms of overperforming adrenals include weight gain, thin skin, high blood sugar, thirst, and extreme emotions.
- Treating overperforming adrenals usually requires surgery.

Other Thyroid-Related Diseases

In This Chapter

- Parathyroid gland problems
- Inflamed thyroid issues
- Thyroid-related tumors
- Thyroid-related eye problems

So far this book has covered hypothyroidism, hyperthyroidism, and cancer. These diseases cause over 95 percent of all thyroid-related problems. However, they aren't the whole story.

Hundreds of thousands of people are diagnosed every year with other thyroid-related illnesses, including parathyroid disease, thyroiditis (inflamed thyroid), thyroid eye disease, and multiple endocrine neoplasia (thyroid tumors).

If you have reason to believe you're suffering from one of these less common conditions, this chapter will provide the information you need for seeking an accurate diagnosis and successful treatment.

Parathyroid Disease

Directly behind your thyroid are small glands, each around the size of a grain of rice, called *parathyroid glands*. There are typically four of them, but the number can vary from person to person.

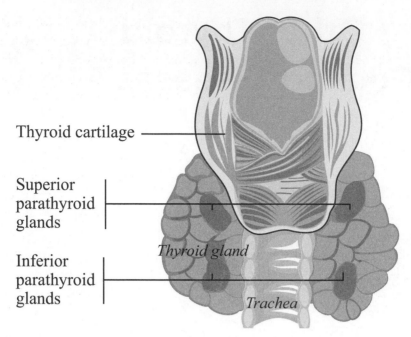

Thyroid cartilage

Superior parathyroid glands

Inferior parathyroid glands

Thyroid gland

Trachea

The parathyroid glands.
(Licensed from Shutterstock Images)

While your parathyroids reside right up against your thyroid, they have an entirely separate function. Their job is to create hormones that regulate the amount of calcium in your blood and bones. That might not sound like a big deal. However, calcium affects such vital functions as preventing your bones from breaking down and transmitting signals to your muscles, which among other things ensures that your heart keeps beating.

Maintaining your calcium levels within the narrow range your body requires (from 8.5 to 10.2 milligrams per deciliter of blood) is a delicate task, so anything that throws your parathyroids off-kilter can result in serious consequences.

There are roughly 100,000 diagnosed cases of parathyroid disease a year in the United States alone. That's around 1 out of every 3,000 people. It's twice as likely to occur in women, and it's six times as likely to occur past age 60.

Parathyroid Disease Causes

One of the most common causes of parathyroid damage is treatment for thyroid disease. That's because the parathyroids are so close to the thyroid.

For example, if a surgeon needs to remove part or all of a thyroid—which is usually the first step in treatment for thyroid cancer, and occasionally for hyperthyroidism—there's a risk the surgeon will accidentally cut one of the parathyroids. This is actually one of the scenarios doctors worry about most when considering thyroid surgery … especially since the precise number, location, and size of parathyroids can be quite different from patient to patient.

Similarly, radiation can be used to either destroy a thyroid's cancer cells or reduce the thyroid's mass to treat hyperthyroidism. Even though the parathyroids aren't being targeted by the radioiodine, there's a risk they'll become damaged simply because of how close they are to the radioactive thyroid cells. In addition, the radiation exposure poses a long-term risk of the parathyroids developing cancer or other dangerous growths themselves.

There are also rare instances in which thyroid disease becomes linked with parathyroid disease. In these cases, someone will have hypothyroidism and her calcium levels will be normal, but once she's treated for the hypothyroidism her latent hyperparathyroid disease will kick in and dangerously increase her calcium.

Parathyroid Disease Symptoms

When something goes wrong with your parathyroids, it can show up as a variety of symptoms. You may sometimes hear these summarized as *bones, stones, and groans.*

Bones refers to when your parathyroids are underperforming by triggering the creation of too little calcium, a condition called *hypoparathyroidism.* Your body responds to this emergency by removing calcium from the place that has the most of it—your bones—so it can keep the calcium levels steady in your bloodstream. That's okay as a short-term solution. However, if calcium continues to be removed from your bones more quickly than it's replaced, your bones will start to break down.

Stones refers to the opposite problem: your parathyroids are overperforming and putting too much calcium in your blood, a condition called *hyperparathyroidism.* This can lead to the calcium turning solid and forming kidney stones.

And *groans* refers to the physical and psychological pain you may feel as your system is disrupted by a calcium imbalance.

As with the thyroid, an ailing parathyroid can result in numerous different symptoms. In general, though, certain symptoms are more likely to occur than others. Take a few minutes to go over this list of common clues to parathyroid malfunction and check off any symptom that applies to you.

Parathyroid Symptoms Checklist

- ❏ Pain in abdomen
- ❏ Pain in muscles
- ❏ Exhaustion
- ❏ Sluggishness
- ❏ Slowed thinking
- ❏ Insomnia
- ❏ Headaches
- ❏ High blood pressure
- ❏ Depression
- ❏ Anxiety
- ❏ Feelings of hostility
- ❏ Obsessive-compulsive behavior
- ❏ Vague sense of not feeling "right"
- ❏ Thinning hair
- ❏ Kidney stones
- ❏ Gastric reflux disease
- ❏ Bone breakdown (e.g., osteoporosis, osteopenia)
- ❏ Back pain
- ❏ Degeneration of the spine
- ❏ Spinal arthritis
- ❏ Heart palpitations
- ❏ Heart attack

If you aren't experiencing at least four of these symptoms, your parathyroids are probably healthy. If you have four or more of these symptoms, however, then you might be suffering from parathyroid disease. If your symptoms are relatively mild, that unfortunately doesn't mean you're at lower risk. There's actually no connection between the severity of parathyroid symptoms and their seriousness. And if left untreated over a long period (e.g., 15 years), parathyroid disease will typically take five years off your life.

Conversely, if you're successfully treated for parathyroid disease, you'll soon experience improvement in *all* your parathyroid-related symptoms. In fact, you're likely to feel better in ways you didn't even expect. That's because some parathyroid problems occur so slowly and subtly that you aren't even aware you have them. Once these symptoms are treated, you'll notice improvements that make you realize you'd been operating at less than 100 percent in a variety of areas. You therefore shouldn't hesitate to check out your symptoms by seeing a doctor.

Diagnosis and Treatment

The good news is that parathyroid disease can be detected—or ruled out—with some simple blood tests. Specifically, your doctor needs to take a small amount of your blood and then order a group of lab tests called a *comprehensive metabolic panel* (also known as a *CMP, chemistry panel, chemistry screen,* or *SMAC test*). These tests are so standard that many doctors perform them on their patients annually as part of a routine checkup. They identify the levels of a variety of critical chemicals in your bloodstream, including calcium.

If it turns out your blood's calcium level, or *serum calcium*, is what it should be, then you don't have a parathyroid problem. If your serum calcium is either too high or too low, though, then there's something wrong. It could be your parathyroids, or it could be something even more serious such as cancer. Your doctor should therefore conduct follow-up blood tests—including one that measures parathyroid hormone output—to hone in on the cause.

CRASH GLANDING

If your doctor fails to identify the reason for your abnormal serum calcium and tells you "Don't worry about it, it's probably nothing," find another doctor who'll do the job right. Considering that possible causes range from parathyroid problems that (if left untreated) can rob years from your life to even deadlier diseases such as cancer, a discovery of serum calcium that's off-kilter should never be ignored.

If it turns out that your body has too much parathyroid hormones—that is, if you have hyperparathyroidism—there are two primary possibilities:

- A single parathyroid gland is generating excess hormones (the situation for roughly 96 percent of patients). In this case, the solution is relatively simple: have an ENT (ear, nose, and throat) surgeon take out that particular defective gland. If you're typical, you'll have three normal parathyroids left, and they'll automatically pick up the slack, producing enough additional hormones to make up for the gland that's been removed.

- All your parathyroids are generating excess hormones (the situation for roughly 4 percent of patients). In this case, you'll be put on permanent medication that reduces your parathyroid hormones to normal levels.

Alternatively, if your body has too little parathyroid hormones—that is, if you have hypoparathyroidism—the treatment is more complicated. You'll need to be put on medication, but also closely monitored to ensure your body's calcium remains at the right levels. Details are beyond the scope of this book, but your doctor will have more information.

Thyroiditis

If your thyroid feels inflamed, you may have *thyroiditis*.

Thyroiditis usually stems from Hashimoto's disease (see Chapter 5). However, there are also several types of thyroiditis that are (usually) temporary illnesses. They include painful subacute thyroiditis, silent thyroiditis, postpartum thyroiditis, and iodine-induced thyroiditis.

Painful Subacute Thyroiditis

Painful subacute thyroiditis (also known as *de Quervain's thyroiditis* or *subacute granulomatous thyroiditis*) typically occurs after a respiratory infection—for example, after you've had the mumps, the flu, or some other virus. If your body's attacks on the virus create high inflammation, that can in turn spawn antibodies that end up attacking your thyroid. If this occurs, you'll probably feel neck pain. If your thyroid swells, you may also have some trouble swallowing or talking. And you may become feverish and weak.

In addition, because nerves can sometimes carry signals of distress beyond the area actually causing the problem, you may feel pain in your ears, jaw, and/or face. Further, you'll become hyperthyroid, which means—among other things—that your heart might start beating too rapidly.

Your doctor can diagnose this condition by giving you an *iodine uptake and thyroid scan.* This involves injecting you with or having you swallow a tiny amount of radioactive iodine, waiting 6-24 hours, and then scanning your neck to get a clear picture of what's going on in your thyroid.

If you have this condition, your doctor should give you a nonsteroidal anti-inflammatory drug—essentially, a prescription-strength equivalent of ibuprofen—to reduce the inflammation. (If that doesn't work, she can alternatively prescribe corticosteroids, which are steroid-based anti-inflammatory drugs.) In addition, your doctor should prescribe beta blockers to prevent your heart from beating too quickly.

With the help of these medications, the chances are good that you'll be okay until the condition clears itself up. However, in rare cases—and especially if the illness is left untreated—the disease can so stress the thyroid that a permanent condition of hypothyroidism results.

Silent Thyroiditis

Silent thyroiditis (also known as *painless thyroiditis* or *subacute lymphocytic thyroiditis*) is another condition in which your body turns on itself by creating antibodies that attack your thyroid.

Unlike painful subacute thyroiditis, this illness isn't spawned by a viral infection; no one knows what causes it. And while it enlarges your thyroid, it doesn't make the thyroid tender and prone to pain.

As with painful subacute thyroiditis, your doctor can diagnose this condition by giving you an iodine uptake and thyroid scan.

If you have silent thyroiditis, you'll start out as hyperthyroid. During this period, your doctor may prescribe beta blockers to prevent your heart from beating too quickly. The hyperthyroidism will typically last for 2-3 months, after which you'll return to normal. You may then become hypothyroid for 2-3 months and require thyroid medication (see Chapter 8). After this phase, your body will probably cure itself, leaving you healthy. In rare cases, though, the thyroid can become so stressed by the illness that it ends up remaining in the hypothyroid state.

Postpartum Thyroiditis

If you're pregnant, your body will make changes to your immune system during and after the pregnancy to ensure the health of both you and your baby. These changes are normally harmless, but 5-7 percent of women spawn antibodies that end up attacking the thyroid. (Most at risk are women with type 1 diabetes.) This typically happens 2-6 months after the baby is born, but can also occur up to a year later. Postpartum thyroiditis can also occur following a miscarriage or an elective abortion, which puts the body through the same kind of immune system changes.

The symptoms, diagnosis, and treatment for postpartum thyroiditis are the same as those for silent thyroiditis. With time and patience, this illness usually rides itself out. For around 20 percent of women, however, the thyroid ends up remaining in a hypothyroid state. And for the other 80 percent, this illness is likely to recur with subsequent pregnancies, and/or as a result of the hormonal changes that come with the onset of menopause.

Iodine-Induced Thyroiditis

For your thyroid to function properly, you need to consume 150-300 micrograms (mcg) of iodine per day. And as long as you don't go over 1,000 mcg (1 milligram) of iodine daily, you're likely to be fine.

If you overdose on iodine, however—for example, by taking an over-the-counter thyroid product that contains iodine megadoses, or by regularly eating a lot of kelp or other iodine-rich seafood—you may get *iodine-induced thyroiditis.* This can also occur if you were on a low-iodine diet for a long time and then abruptly switch to a normal intake of iodine. In either case, you're shocking your thyroid into processing more iodine than it's accustomed to.

The problem is that as much as 45 percent of people are estimated to have latent thyroid disease—that is, antibodies floating around for Hashimoto's disease or Graves' disease that normally don't do any harm. But when your thyroid is disrupted by an abrupt change in iodine, or by steady iodine megadoses, this can trigger the antibodies into actively attacking your thyroid. As a result, you'll suddenly become hypothyroid or hyperthyroid.

The simple solution is to stop taking the excess iodine. In many cases, your body will heal and you'll become healthy again. However, it may be that once the thyroid disease is triggered, it becomes permanent. If this happens, you'll need to be treated for either hypothyroidism (see Chapter 8) or hyperthyroidism (see Chapter 12), depending on your condition.

Thyroid Eye Disease

If you have Graves' disease—or, more rarely, Hashimoto's disease—there's a chance the same type of antibodies attacking your thyroid will enlarge your eye cells and ocular tissues.

Symptoms you might feel in your eyes include:

- Continual pain, or pain when looking around
- Dryness or itchiness
- Double vision or other impaired vision
- Bloodshot eyes
- Inflammation and swelling
- Swelling in the orbital tissues

The latter can cause your eyeball to push forward, creating a wide-eyed, bulging look.

The usual treatments are eye drops and ointments to ease suffering until the disease goes away.

Thyroid eye disease can subside for a while and then return. If it disappears for more than six months, it's usually gone for good. For about 3 percent of patients who have thyroid eye disease, however, the disease won't end by itself. In these cases, surgery is required.

Also, even if the disease disappears on its own, the wide-eyed look can sometimes remain. When this happens, surgery is required to restore the eyes to normal.

MEN Syndrome

Around 1 out of every 30,000 people has a genetic defect called *multiple endocrine neoplasia 1*, or *MEN1* (also known as *Werner's Syndrome*); or *multiple endocrine neoplasia 2*, or *MEN2* (also known as *Sipple's Syndrome*).

MEN1 causes several different endocrine glands—the thyroid, parathyroids, pancreas, pituitary, and/or adrenals—to start growing tumors at the same time. These tumors usually aren't cancerous. But the enlargements of the glands leads to an overproduction of hormones. This can show up as a wide variety of symptoms—headaches, blurred vision, racing heartbeat, and scores of other possibilities—because these glands affect almost every area of your body. Left untreated, the excess hormones can severely damage your quality of life, and even take years off your life.

MEN1 runs in families, and it can be detected through gene testing. It can also be diagnosed through blood tests checking hormone levels. There's currently no cure for MEN1. However, once detected, the tumors it creates can be removed via surgery, or the excess hormones can be suppressed via medication.

MEN2 is similar to MEN1 in that it causes endocrine glands to grow tumors. Unfortunately, with MEN2 the tumors are usually cancerous. That means they can spread from the glands to other parts of your body, which makes them deadly.

MEN2 also runs in families and can be detected through gene testing. If you're unlucky enough to win this genetic lottery, you should be closely monitored. If or when cancerous tumors occur, they can be destroyed using surgery and/or radiation.

The Least You Need to Know

- Get a comprehensive metabolic panel blood test annually to check your calcium levels; and if they're abnormal, be sure to identify the cause.

- Avoid iodine megadoses and abrupt increases in iodine consumption.

- If your eyes have been bothering you for no reason, or if you recently gave birth, get your blood tested for thyroid antibodies.

- If your family has a history of multiple endocrine neoplasia (MEN), get your genes tested.

Emotions and Your Thyroid

Chapter 16

In This Chapter

- Understanding how chemicals affect emotions
- Taking depression and anxiety seriously
- Using T3 to fight depression
- Mood swings and antibody testing
- The thyroid's role in bipolar disorder

One of the worst aspects of thyroid disease is the havoc it can play with our minds and emotions. The physical symptoms of a thyroid problem (such as gaining weight or losing hair) are easy to spot. Mental symptoms such as clinical depression or anxiety are more subtle ... and more likely to be dismissed as being the result of stress, personal issues, or "just your imagination."

However, they're very real illnesses. Millions of people struggle with mental disorders, and many of them could be cured if they simply realized the source of their pain was an easily treatable thyroid condition.

How Hormones Rule Us

The relationship between our intangible minds and physical bodies has been a topic of conjecture and wonder for ages. While no one understands all the nuances of the mind-body connection, it's undeniable that your thoughts and moods are heavily influenced by the "chemical soup" that's constantly circulating in your blood and interacting with your brain. And among the chemicals that have the biggest impact are your hormones.

If you're a woman, you know how enormously moods can be affected by the hormonal upheavals that accompany PMS, menstruation, pregnancy, post-pregnancy, and menopause.

And if you're a man, think back to when you became an adolescent and your thoughts suddenly started focusing on sex, and you became more aggressive. Also recall that as you grew older, your sex drive became less urgent and your attitude mellowed. These changes were orchestrated by your hormones.

More specifically, each cell in your body has multiple mini-programs built into it called *receptors*. When a hormone designed to generate a particular activity enters a cell containing a receptor for that activity, the hormone behaves like the ignition key in an engine and turns on the receptor. The cell then performs the appropriate action.

When it comes to thyroid hormones, among the activities that can be activated are energy production, cell growth, and the manufacturing of critical chemicals. That might not sound significant within the context of one tiny cell, but your brain is composed of *billions* of cells. When hormones activate a large number of receptors in your brain at the same time, the emotional effects can be overwhelming.

Unfortunately, the same holds true when brain cells that would normally be activated suddenly aren't—for example, due to a hormone shortage caused by hypothyroidism. The painful numbness of this lack of activity has been described by some depressed patients as "the void."

Many people feel embarrassed or ashamed about having a disease that impacts their emotions. In the past there's been a terrible lack of understanding about such illnesses, and a tendency to blame those who have them. Given what medical science now knows about these problems, however, there should be no more of a stigma associated with depression or anxiety than there is with having asthma or diabetes. All these conditions are the result of something gone wrong with the body's internal chemistry—and they're all treatable.

Diagnosing and Treating Depression

If you're hypothyroid, one of the results of your brain having an insufficient amount of T3 can be clinical depression. While the cause is straightforward—your brain isn't being supplied with the energy it needs—the consequences can be devastating. As many who've suffered this illness will attest, almost nothing compares to its special kind of pain.

THROAT QUOTE

I once went to a psychiatrist and I said, "I'll do anything, get me out of this." And he said, "I know what you're going through. When one of my parents died, I went through awful grief."

"Do you think grief is anything like depression?" I told him.

Go with the grief, it's better. In grief, you're at least feeling a rich, deep feeling. In depression, you don't even have that. It's just that awful drone of nullity.

—TV host/author Dick Cavett, speaking about his depression

People who've never experienced clinical depression often mistake it for no more than sadness, and their response may be to tell you to "get over it" or "cheer up." That's like suggesting to someone with cancer to "just tell your cells to be healthy again." A more pragmatic approach is needed.

The good news is if your depression stems entirely from a lack of thyroid hormone, taking thyroid medication should soon cure it. This is often so effective that it can seem like magic. However, the medication is simply providing your brain with the chemicals it needs to function properly.

One qualification is that taking T4 alone—for example, in the form of Synthroid—might not be effective. No one is sure why, but when it comes to depression what typically works best is taking T3 directly (as opposed to relying on your body to convert T4 to T3). Therefore, taking any of the following is likely to work:

- Desiccated thyroid (such as Nature-Throid), which is a natural mix of T4 and T3.

- A mix of Synthroid (synthetic T4) and Cytomel (synthetic T3).

- A mix of desiccated thyroid and Synthroid. This can make sense when you need a T4-to-T3 ratio that can't be achieved with desiccated thyroid alone.

If your only problem was an underperforming thyroid, then once you're on the right hormone dosage—and especially the right amount of direct T3—your depression should disappear. If your depression lifts to a degree but doesn't go away, then there could be causes for it beyond your thyroid. In this case you should keep taking T3, but in addition pursue other treatments such as exercise, talk therapy, and/or anti-depressant medication.

For the latter, you can have your doctor prescribe a conventional antidepressant such as Zoloft, Paxil, or Prozac. Alternatively, you can try natural medicines that raise serotonin levels such as tryptophan and 5-HTP (which are available over-the-counter, but it's best to adjust their dosages under a doctor's supervision).

THYROIDIAN TIP

It's fine to mix antidepressants and T3. In fact, many doctors use T3 as a supplement to antidepressants even when there's no evidence of a thyroid problem. Although no one knows why, T3 frequently helps alleviate or cure the depression. In such cases what's prescribed is Cytomel—or its generic version liothyronine—which is the only medication available that's pure T3 (as opposed to a T4/T3 mix). As long as free T3 levels are monitored via periodic blood tests (to avoid overdosing and hyperthyroidism), there's no downside to giving T3 a chance when conventional antidepressants have failed.

Diagnosing and Treating Anxiety

Anxiety is a frequent symptom of hyperthyroidism. As your metabolism speeds up, you're likely to become more tense, nervous, and apprehensive about everyday events for no apparent reason. In addition, your heart may beat exceptionally fast, making you feel as if you drank a pot of coffee.

Victims of anxiety often blame their feelings on stress; but if you weren't anxious previously and nothing notable has changed in your life, it's wise to get tested for a physical cause—including an overactive thyroid.

 THROAT QUOTE

Anxiety is the rust of life, destroying its brightness and weakening its power.

—Anonymous

Paradoxically, anxiety can also stem from Hashimoto's disease, which is the primary cause of *hypo*thyroidism.

That's because Hashimoto's breaks down the colloid cells that make up your thyroid. The destruction of these cells progressively shrinks your thyroid until it's unable to produce the amount of hormones you need. During the early stages of Hashimoto's, however, every time a bunch of colloid cells are ruptured they release the thyroid hormones they were storing. This abrupt spurt of extra hormones into your body can make you temporarily hyperthyroid—which may result in feelings of anxiousness, nervousness, and/or irritability. Over time you'll feel a gradual decline in hormones as your body returns to normal, and as your thyroid works at reduced capacity. But then the Hashimoto's will strike again, and you'll undergo another episode of hyperthyroidism.

This cycle of highs and lows—which is called *Hashitoxicosis*—is likely to create wild mood swings. If your doctor tests your TSH, T4, and T3 levels, however, they might all show up as normal, because the highs and lows often end up balancing each other out. Unless your doctor happens to take your blood during a period when the Hashimoto's is attacking and your thyroid levels are spiking, standard blood tests may label your thyroid as functioning perfectly.

To account for this, your first blood workup should additionally cover antibodies. Since Hashimoto's is an autoimmune disease, it'll be detected via tests for antibodies attacking your thyroid, at which point your doctor can take a closer look via an ultrasound.

It's actually a good idea to check for antibodies in *any* initial thyroid blood testing. Nonetheless, most doctors neglect this step. So if you're experiencing mood swings, insist that antibody testing be included in your doctor's orders to the lab.

If it turns out your anxiety is being caused by standard hyperthyroidism—for example, the autoimmune disorder Graves' disease—then see Chapter 12 for information on treatment options.

If the cause is Hashitoxicosis, however, then your doctor will prescribe anti-anxiety medication to allow you to "ride out" the periodic attacks. Over time the Hashimoto's will stabilize, putting you into a permanent hypothyroid state that can be managed easily with thyroid pills (see Chapters 8 and 9).

> **THYROIDIAN TIP**
>
> No one knows why, but anxiety can also be a symptom of standard hypothyroidism. This isn't as common as anxiety stemming from an overactive thyroid, but it happens. So if you're diagnosed as having low thyroid activity and you feel anxiety, it's not your imagination; and the problem will probably go away once you're on thyroid medication.

Other Mental Disorders

Thyroid symptoms can resemble a wide range of mental problems beyond depression and anxiety. For example, if you're hypothyroid, you may become foggy and confused, and have memory lapses that resemble Alzheimer's disease (such as forgetting if it's summer or winter). But while Alzheimer's is incurable and fatal, hypothyroidism can be readily managed with medication. This is especially a problem for the elderly, as roughly 25 percent of people age 75 and over are estimated to be hypothyroid; but their thyroid-related symptoms will often be misdiagnosed as age-related dementia and go untreated.

As another example, if you're severely hyperthyroid you may experience hallucinations, delusions, and other symptoms associated with psychosis. Patients are periodically misdiagnosed as suffering from schizophrenia when they just have an overactive thyroid.

Then again, hyperthyroidism might lead you to become manic—for example, impulsive, reckless, or promiscuous, and skipping sleep for days on end until your body gives out and you "crash." If the hormone spike is due to a Hashimoto's attack, then soon afterward you're likely to swing down the other direction into depression. This high/low cycle can easily be mistaken for bipolar disorder.

A particularly insidious complication with bipolar disorder is that many of the medications used to treat it—especially the newer ones, such as carbamazepine and Depakote—have side effects that include weight gain, depression, dry skin, hair loss … in other words, signs of hypothyroidism. So if your onset of Hashimoto's is mistaken for bipolar disorder, and you go on to develop full-blown hypothyroidism, it'll be almost impossible to tell from your symptoms; your doctor will just assume you're experiencing the side effects of the bipolar drugs. There are patients who needlessly suffered for years for just this reason.

Considering that thyroid disease symptoms can so closely mimic both those of mental illnesses and the side effects of medications used to treat them, a wise precaution when seeing a doctor for the first time about a mental issue is to insist on having thyroid blood tests done—including antibody tests. You may find that your problems are stemming entirely from your thyroid.

Alternatively, you might really have the mental illness your symptoms indicate—but *also* have a thyroid problem that's making it *even worse*. For example, if you have bipolar disorder, and in addition have even a slight leaning toward hypothyroidism, the latter may make you resistant to the mood stabilizers used to treat the bipolar condition. Doctors who understand this will put you on thyroid medication and adjust the dosage until your T4 and T3 levels are as perfect as possible. (This is analogous to adding T3 to antidepressants; even if your lab tests show your thyroid to be normal, the added hormones can make your medication more effective.)

One other nasty complication with bipolar disease is that one of its treatments, lithium, is chemically close enough to iodine to be eagerly absorbed by your thyroid. Over time, there's a greater than 30 percent chance this will damage your thyroid and lead to hypothyroidism. Because of this, lithium is seldom the first choice for treating bipolar disorder. For some people, however, lithium works better than anything else. If that applies to you, have your doctor check your thyroid every 2-3 months to make sure it's remaining healthy despite the risk posed by the medication.

The Least You Need to Know

- Millions of people are suffering needlessly from mental problems that can be cured with or helped by thyroid medication.
- Clinical depression and anxiety are real illnesses caused by chemical imbalances … and nothing to ashamed of.

- T3 is a powerful tool against depression, either by itself or working with antidepressant medication.
- If you have anxiety, ask your doctor to run thyroid antibody blood tests, because you could have a form of thyroid disease that doesn't show up on a standard TSH test.

For Women Only

In This Chapter

- PMS symptoms interacting with hypothyroidism
- Thyroid-related causes of infertility
- Preventing a thyroid-related miscarriage
- Managing thyroid ills during perimenopause

If you're a woman, you're over five times as likely to develop thyroid disease as a man. Your chances of being struck by a thyroid disorder at some point in your life may be as high as 20 percent.

You also have special challenges that men don't. For example, going through hormonal upheavals such as PMS and menopause isn't fun even under normal circumstances; but having thyroid disease will make such tough times substantially worse. And if you're having trouble getting pregnant, you should be aware that hypothyroidism might be preventing it from happening.

This chapter covers the special impact thyroid disease has on women. In most cases, treatment is quick and easy—as long as you're empowered with the knowledge of how to recognize a thyroid-related problem and manage it.

PMS

If you have premenstrual syndrome, you're far from alone. PMS has been estimated to affect over 85 percent of women between the ages of 20 and 40. While PMS symptoms are no picnic even when you're healthy, they can magnify when combined with thyroid issues.

To appreciate why, you first need to understand what's happening in your body during your monthly cycle. After you comprehend the causes of PMS and how they interact with thyroid symptoms, you may find that thyroid medication coupled with simple over-the-counter remedies help enormously.

THROAT QUOTE

Just before their periods, women behave the way men do all the time.

—Robert Heinlein

Understanding PMS

If you're typical, your period lasts 3-5 days. If we count the first day of bleeding as day 1, then ovulation occurs on days 10-15; and your whole cycle lasts 28-30 days.

Your ovaries produce two primary hormones, *estrogen* and *progesterone*. They'll begin secreting estrogen a day or two before ovulation. After that your estrogen level will go down for a while, and then reach its highest levels during days 17-23. Progesterone isn't made during the first half of the cycle, but is secreted right after ovulation, and then maintained at high levels during days 16-25. That means both estrogen and progesterone are operating in force during days 17-23, with their peak around day 21.

These hormones travel through your entire body, first targeting your brain, your breasts, and your uterus. They then recirculate and go to your liver, where they get bound up by carrier proteins (mostly *glucuronic acid*) and are then sent through the bile into your colon. If all goes well, these hormones then leave your body via the stool.

But what often happens during peak hormone production—around day 21—is a certain amount of hormones escape the liver, or become loosened from their carrier proteins in the colon, and reenter your bloodstream. They'll then circulate around your body again. As they do, by-products from these "used" hormones have negative effects on your brain's chemistry. For example, they can make you feel depressed, anxious, angry, or edgy; make you foggy and forgetful; and lead to mood swings and crying spells. They can also make you crave sugar and/or salt.

The by-products can additionally affect your breasts, making them enlarged and tender. And they can thicken the uterine lining, making it harder to push out through the cervix, which leads to menstrual pain and cramps. These hormones with bad by-products will then return to your liver and colon; but they might escape and recirculate one or two more times before finally exiting your body. The problems they cause are a large reason why you feel uncomfortable a week or so before your period.

Another factor is that the hormones moving through the colon change the colon's chemistry. This can cause nausea, upset stomach, gas, bloating, irregularity, constipation, and/or diarrhea. The high level of hormones can also raise the background level of inflammation in the body, leading to backaches, headaches, and joint and muscle pain.

On top of all that, estrogen blocks T3 from entering your cells' membranes. This means when you have more estrogen in your system, fewer cells in your body can make use of available thyroid hormones.

If your thyroid is working normally, you'll simply ride out the third week in your cycle when estrogen is peaking and keeping you from receiving the full benefit of available T3. But if you're already on the verge of hypothyroidism—if your thyroid is subtly underperforming, or if you're on thyroid medication but the dosage is too low—then hypothyroid symptoms are likely to become prominent. These include fatigue, insomnia, acne, weight gain, and more (see Chapter 6). They also include symptoms you might already be accustomed to as a result of recycled hormones affecting your brain chemistry, such as depression, anxiety, and mood swings. However, the lack of adequate T3 can make what might otherwise be mild problems into major ones.

These ills can be difficult to recognize as thyroid related because they're common aspects of PMS. But if you're experiencing an abrupt increase in their severity, or notice symptoms that have never happened before, then don't hesitate to get your thyroid tested.

THYROIDIAN TIP

When you get your blood taken for thyroid testing, be sure to tell your doctor where you're at in your cycle. That's because if you're in week three (when your hormones are peaking), your TSH level will be artificially raised a bit, making it appear higher than it really is the rest of the month. An experienced doctor will know this and take it into account when evaluating your test results.

Managing PMS

If testing reveals you're hypothyroid, then the most effective way you can reduce your PMS symptoms is by starting on thyroid medication. In addition, there are some simple things you can do to help your body prevent "used" estrogen hormones escaping from your liver or colon to re-circulate and spread unhealthy byproducts.

First, cut down on coffee, because caffeine helps estrogen escape the liver. It's also helpful to reduce *methylxanthines*, which are caffeine-like substances contained in chocolate and cocoa products.

Next, during the third week of your cycle when estrogen is peaking, consider taking 500 milligrams a day of *calcium d-glucarate*. This is an over-the-counter version of glucuronic acid, which is the protein your body uses to bind estrogen and keep it from leaving your colon. Calcium d-glucarate has virtually no side effects; and increasing your body's supply of glucuronic acid when it needs it most will help ensure the used estrogen stays in your colon until your body is ready to evict it via the stool.

CRASH GLANDING

When you look for calcium d-glucarate, don't mistakenly buy calcium glucanate. While their names are very similar, they're entirely different chemically and have entirely different effects.

You should also get more fiber in your colon. Fiber creates helpful bacteria that degrade used hormones into harmless chemicals (and, as a nice side effect, lower long-term risks of breast and ovarian cancer). Ideal for this purpose is *ground flax seed*, which you can find in any health food store. Sprinkling a couple of tablespoons a day on top of cereal, smoothies, or soup during the third week of your cycle should do the trick. It's best to spread out the two tablespoons over a few meals instead of consuming it all at once, though; otherwise you may feel gassy and bloated until your body gets used to the ground flax seed.

In addition, take calcium during your third week—specifically, 1,300-1,500 milligrams per day of *calcium citrate* or *calcium citrate malate*. These calcium supplements help to inhibit hormone byproducts from acting on your brain cells.

If you're experiencing significant aches, pains, and cramping, over-the-counter anti-inflammatories such as ibuprofen and naproxen sodium are fine for most people, as long as they're used short-term and at the recommended doses.

More generally, living healthy makes a big difference (see Part 5). Choose a balanced and nutritious diet, exercise regularly, get enough sleep, and engage in relaxing activities like spending time with friends. The stronger your body and mind are, the less vulnerable you'll be to hormonal byproducts.

Further, maintain a steady level of blood sugar. For example, don't skip meals, and eat balanced portions at each meal. Otherwise your adrenal glands may produce extra cortisol (see Chapter 14), and that can add to the hormonal havoc of PMS.

If all these relatively simple measures aren't enough, though, you can additionally turn to your doctor for help.

For example, most PMS problems are caused by high levels of estrogen, while progesterone serves to block estrogen. If you're between 35 and 45, there's a chance your ovaries are secreting less progesterone, which means your body is effectively dealing with more estrogen, heightening your PMS. It's a bad idea to self-medicate progesterone because it's not always needed, and it has significant side effects; but you can ask a doctor who's an expert on PMS to check your hormone levels when you're around day 21 of your cycle and, if appropriate, prescribe a relevant dosage of progesterone for you.

Finally, if your PMS makes you depressed and taking T3 doesn't entirely resolve it, you can ask your doctor to additionally prescribe an antidepressant. For example, there's a PMS-specific version of Prozac designed to be used only during the third week of each cycle.

If a thyroid problem is underlying your PMS issues, there's a good chance taking thyroid medication and following at least some of the solutions just described will allow you to live relatively happily with your PMS.

Infertility

One of life's most precious gifts is our ability to have children. And so one of the most heartbreaking ailments is the seeming inability to become pregnant. Fertility problems sometimes stem from genetics or from age. But they're also often brought about by thyroid disease, which is easily treatable.

Hypothyroidism can cause infertility in a number of ways. First, thyroid hormones—and particularly T3—regulate the rate of cell growth. If your body doesn't have enough T3, it can inhibit the formation of the cells that support the egg, or *ovum*. A telltale sign of this occurring is irregular cycles.

Low T3 can also inhibit the production of progesterone, a hormone critical for ovulation. If this happens, your periods may stop altogether.

Another reason for infertility is a hormone called *prolactin*, which your body normally produces after you give birth to make your breasts lactate. Prolactin inhibits a sperm's ability to enter an egg, making it unlikely (though not impossible) that you'll get pregnant while nursing your newborn baby.

When your thyroid is underactive, your pituitary gland will release more TSH to stimulate the production of thyroid hormones. By coincidence, the pituitary is also in charge of making prolactin, and sometimes when it's churning out an unusually large amount of TSH, it'll inappropriately churn out prolactin, too.

In fact, having a high level of prolactin is one of the first noticeable signs of early thyroid disease. There usually won't be enough prolactin to make you lactate, but it could cause your periods to abruptly stop. And even if the latter doesn't occur, the prolactin will vastly decrease your chances of getting pregnant. Once you treat your hypothyroidism, though, your pituitary gland will stop making excessive TSH—and will simultaneously quit secreting prolactin.

Miscarriage

As painful as infertility is, even more tragic is a miscarriage. Unfortunately, thyroid problems greatly increase this risk, especially during the first trimester.

That's because for the first nine weeks your baby can't make thyroid hormones, and so must rely entirely on your own T4 and T3. If your thyroid underproduces its hormones during this time and you don't take medication to correct the imbalance, it can severely impair your baby's development.

Further, if your hypothyroidism is caused by an autoimmune response, the increase in roving antibodies seeking foreign invaders to attack poses an additional danger to your baby.

It's common to be mildly hypothyroid before becoming pregnant and not be aware of it. It's also common to be latently hypothyroid—that is, have no symptoms at all, but be on the verge of thyroid disease. In either case, the upheaval of hormones that comes with pregnancy can nudge a thyroid from being barely healthy to ailing.

Pregnancy also brings vast changes to your immune system (because your body suddenly has to take into account not only your health but the health of your baby). As these transformations occur, they can spawn antibodies that attack both your thyroid and the thyroid hormones circulating in your blood, putting you into a hypothyroid state.

To make matters worse, hypothyroidism is far from obvious during pregnancy, because many of its symptoms—such as weight gain, fatigue, mood swings, and insomnia—can be attributed to the pregnancy itself.

Therefore, if you're pregnant, it's important for your doctor to test your thyroid (including antibody testing) as soon as your condition is known, and at least every 2-3 months after that.

If your thyroid is healthy, no harm is done in checking it. But if it's started under-performing, then thyroid medication will quickly get your T3 level back to where it needs to be; and it'll also lower your TSH level, which is likely to reduce antibody activity. This helps ensure your pregnancy remains on course.

Alternatively, you could become hyperthyroid during pregnancy. This is much less common; it happens only about 1 percent of the time. The main dangers are an increased heart rate for both you and your baby; a quicker metabolism, which can impair your body's ability to deliver sufficient nourishment to the baby; and a surplus of thyroid hormones, which will do you no harm but poses a risk for your still-developing child. Since neither radiation nor anti-thyroid medications are safe for your baby, the best option for this situation is generally surgery to reduce your thyroid's size. If the result is an underactive thyroid, you can then take medication to get your thyroid hormone levels back to normal.

Postpartum Problems

Virtually everyone knows that a woman's body goes through massive hormonal and immune system changes during pregnancy. What not so many people consider is that it goes through similar transformations after giving birth. The conditions the body operated under for nine months no longer apply, and so it has to make major adjustments.

For example, there are very high levels of the hormone progesterone during pregnancy, which helps thyroid hormones enter cells efficiently and so lowers the amount of work the thyroid has to do. After birth, however, there's an enormous drop in progesterone levels. This puts an abrupt and heavy strain on the thyroid, which all of a sudden needs to produce substantially more hormones than it was accustomed to for the previous nine months. This shock can trigger either a temporary or permanent thyroid problem.

One result is an autoimmune disorder called Graves' disease (see Chapter 10). The good news is there are more options for managing hyperthyroidism after pregnancy than during it (see Chapter 12).

A disease that so frequently occurs after birth that it takes its name from it is *postpartum thyroiditis* (see Chapter 15). Because this is an autoimmune disease, antibody testing is especially important to detect it. This illness tends to end automatically after several months, and in the meantime is quite treatable; the trick is diagnosing it before a great deal of unnecessary suffering takes place.

Most common of all is hypothyroidism. This can cause unrelenting postpartum depression, as well as other severe symptoms. As terrible as its effects can be, however, it's the most easily treatable of these thyroid conditions (see Chapters 8 and 9).

During the first six months after you give birth, you'll be faced with numerous challenges: learning to be a good parent, dealing with lack of sleep, and becoming a magician at juggling multiple tasks. It's normal to feel physically run down and emotionally exhausted from it all. But if you're suffering from thyroid disease on top of that, you'll feel much worse than any mother should have to. If you suspect your thyroid is malfunctioning, don't hesitate to see your doctor. A simple blood test and some inexpensive pills may spare you from awful symptoms during what should be the happiest time of your life.

Perimenopause and Menopause

Unlike thyroid disease, diagnosing menopause couldn't be more straightforward. There are no lab tests involved, and only one relevant symptom: whether you've had any periods over the past 12 months.

If you have, but your periods have been increasingly intermittent over time, then you're in *perimenopause*. This is a long-term stage during which your sex hormones—first *androgen* (which influences your sex drive and energy level), then progesterone, and finally estrogen—are steadily declining.

Specifically, around ages 38-42 your androgen levels significantly lower. This typically dampens your libido, slows your metabolic rate, and causes a general feeling of fatigue. It can also diminish the growth of lean body mass, forcing you to exercise more to avoid gaining fat (even as it makes you feel less energetic about exercising).

Around ages 42-45 progesterone levels decrease, which usually makes your PMS symptoms more severe and alters the timing of your cycles (causing you to miss periods, or at the other extreme experience mid-cycle bleeding).

Around ages 45-47 estrogen levels go down. The lessening stimulus of the uterine lining to thicken itself and cause your cycle to occur eventually leads to your periods stopping. It's during this phase that you start experiencing night sweats and hot flashes.

Your last menstrual cycle typically occurs within a few months of your fiftieth birthday (though if it happens a few years earlier or later, that's perfectly normal, too). And a year after that, you're officially in menopause.

All these phases involve major changes to your body's hormone activity, and that opens the door to your thyroid becoming strained and defective. When you consider the odds of getting thyroid disease go up with age anyway, it's understandable that many women become hypothyroid at some point during perimenopause.

Unfortunately, the hypothyroidism is often missed by doctors, because its key symptoms—weight gain, fatigue, and depression—can be attributed to perimenopause-related changes. That means it's your job to keep a special eye out for thyroid symptoms during this time of your life. If you have any reason to suspect hypothyroidism, see your doctor and get tested.

And even if you don't notice any symptoms, it's a good idea to get tested as part of your annual checkup once you begin perimenopause. Having a baseline reading on your thyroid hormone levels will make it easier for you and your doctor to later notice subtle indications that your thyroid is starting to underperform. If your T4 and T3 levels remain normal but your TSH begins creeping up, try following the advice in Chapters 18 and 22; it may help you avoid progressing into hypothyroidism.

The Least You Need to Know

- If your PMS symptoms are severe, get your thyroid tested to learn whether it's making a tough time worse.
- If you're experiencing trouble getting pregnant, have your doctor check your thyroid.
- Get tested for thyroid disease as soon as you learn you're pregnant, and then every 2-3 months during the pregnancy.
- Get tested for thyroid disease—including antibody testing—within a few months of giving birth.
- Get tested for thyroid disease as part of your annual checkup from around age 38 on.

Diet and Lifestyle

This final part explains that medicine isn't the only way to improve your thyroid. Eating the right foods, avoiding artificial chemicals and toxins, and minimizing stress play important roles as well.

And in case you gained weight while you were hypothyroid, Chapters 19 and 20 offer expert advice on how to shed both pounds and fat.

Eating Your Way to Health

In This Chapter

- Cutting down on processed foods
- Minimizing pesticides and food toxins
- Going organic
- Matching foods to your metabolism

Medication isn't the only way to ensure your health. At least as important is making smart choices about what you eat every day. Foods that are free of toxins, and that work well with your metabolic rate, are especially good for your thyroid … and for your body overall.

If you don't yet have a thyroid problem, or are in just a mild early stage, changing your food habits for the better may help prevent your thyroid from getting worse. Conversely, if you're already suffering from thyroid disease, what you eat might help heal and strengthen your thyroid. This chapter will therefore provide advice on what foods to seek out and what to avoid.

Choosing Natural vs. Processed Foods

As explained in Chapter 5, your thyroid is especially sensitive to artificial chemicals and toxins. The more of them you consume, the more they're likely to accumulate in your thyroid and make it malfunction. It's therefore always a good idea to favor fresh, natural foods over processed foods.

First, the processing of the food may involve harmful chemicals. For example, it was recently discovered that some manufacturers of corn syrup use mercury-based components, resulting in small amounts of mercury turning up in thousands of snacks, beverages, and other foods that include corn syrup in their ingredients.

Mercury is poisonous to the entire body, but it's especially harmful to the thyroid because it's chemically similar to iodine. That means your thyroid will absorb any mercury in your bloodstream and store it. Even though the amount in any one serving of food is minute, over time the mercury can accumulate to a level where it attracts the attention of your immune system and triggers a thyroid autoimmune disease such as Hashimoto's or Graves'.

If that scenario seems far-fetched, consider that corn growing is heavily government subsidized in the United States, making corn syrup exceptionally inexpensive … and included in just about every type of processed food imaginable. So if you're straying from natural foods, your daily intake of corn syrup—and bits of mercury—may be a lot higher than you realize.

And beyond the toxins that are accidentally included in processed food, you have to worry about the chemicals that are included intentionally.

Our air, water, offices, and homes are filled with artificial chemicals—there are over 100,000 registered for commercial use in the United States alone.

Many of these substances haven't been around long enough for us to know what their long-term effects will be. Just as importantly, no one knows how you'll be affected by the combination of hundreds of chemicals in your daily life that have never been tested together.

So when you check the ingredients label of a processed food and see chemicals listed that no one's grandmother ever heard of, let alone would make a welcome part of a homemade meal, be aware that consuming that food is gambling with the health of both your thyroid and your whole body.

THYROIDIAN TIP

If you don't like reading labels, employ this rule of thumb: Glance at a food's list of ingredients. If it's a long list, the food is probably loaded with chemicals … and you should return it to the shelf.

Avoiding Toxins in Produce

Even if you stick to natural foods you're not home free, because artificial chemicals and toxins are all around us. For example, mainstream farms use a substantial amount of pesticides to keep insects from devouring the food being grown. The levels of the toxins are supposed to be safe for humans, but no one really knows what their long-term effects will be on us.

The simplest solution is to eat organic produce. These are fruits and vegetables grown the old-fashioned way, with no artificial chemicals or poisons. Added benefits are that such produce is richer in nutrients and tastes better.

While organic produce tends to be more expensive, you can typically find bargains via local family farms and farmers' markets. Two great resources for finding these are the websites Local Harvest (LocalHarvest.org) and USDA Agricultural Marketing Service (Apps.ams.usda.gov/FarmersMarkets).

Another simple technique is to buy seasonably and flexibly. For example, if the peaches you want are priced sky-high in a given week but mangos are on sale, consider buying the mangos instead. Making such on-the-spot substitutions can save you a bundle. (It can even help your health, since seasonal fruit is typically fresher and so contains more antioxidants.)

Then again, you can mix mainstream and organic produce strategically. For example, fruit with hard skins that you discard—such as bananas and watermelons—are less likely to be affected by pesticides, so you can opt to buy those from conventional retailers. However, when it comes to produce that's typically soaked in pesticides—such as strawberries and spinach—consider paying more for the organic versions.

Also high in pesticides are peanuts and raisins. Especially if you tend to feed these to your kids as snacks, buy the organic versions.

THYROIDIAN TIP

To access lists of fruits and vegetables that tend to have the highest and lowest levels of pesticides, visit this book's website at www.CIGThyroid.com.

Avoiding Toxins in Meat

Even more worrisome sources of toxins are beef, pork, poultry, and fish. That's because the higher you go up the food chain, the more likely it is that an animal consumed toxins and is then passing them along to you when you eat that animal.

For example, modern farms often feed their animals corn—again, because corn is government subsidized in the U.S. and so is very inexpensive. The corn has pesticides that the cows end up consuming and storing in their bodies.

A related problem is that cows were never designed to eat corn, so their intestinal tracts quickly form toxic *E. coli* bacteria. Farmers therefore also feed the cows antibiotics to kill the *E. coli*, and loading up on those isn't good for you, either.

On top of all that, roughly two thirds of beef cows in the U.S. are fed recombinant bovine growth hormone (rBGH) to make them reach their slaughter weight faster. These hormones are stored in their bodies and passed along to you. There's such concern about this practice that Canada, the European Union, Japan, and Australia have banned rBGH and no longer import beef from the United States.

The safest approach when it comes to meat—aside from becoming a vegetarian—is, once again, to buy organic. For example, cows raised naturally on grass rather than corn won't be stuffed with antibiotics or pesticides; and they won't be fed rBGH, either. In addition, such cows will end up producing leaner meat, with higher-quality fats (such as omega-3 fats, which are good for you)—and will be substantially tastier.

While organic meat is more expensive, you may score deals via local family farms and ranches. To locate pasture-based farms near you that sell grass-fed meat and dairy products, visit the website Eatwild.com.

If buying organic isn't convenient or affordable, though, you can at least minimize the amount of toxins you're eating by avoiding the animal's fat. That's because toxins tend to get stored in the fat. So buying lean meat, cutting away fat, removing skin, favoring white meat over dark, and so on will reduce your exposure to the unhealthy chemicals that animals consume.

Foods Fitting Your Metabolism

Another way to eat smart is to be aware of which foods are a good fit for your metabolic rate (see Chapter 1). If you're hypothyroid, your insulin will be less effective at lowering blood sugar and helping convert it into energy. You'll therefore want to eat foods that can put your body into "calorie burning mode" rather than "food storage mode."

For example, high-fiber fruits and vegetables (peaches, broccoli, carrots), legumes (pinto beans, chickpeas, lentils), and high-protein foods (white meat poultry, cottage cheese, soy products) will stay in your stomach for a while before moving on to your small intestines, and then your bloodstream. This allows for gradual digestion and low releases of blood sugar, requiring relatively little insulin; and it puts your body into a "calorie burning mode" that's likely to turn the food directly into energy.

Conversely, sugary low-fiber foods (cookies, donuts) and starchy foods (potatoes, pasta) speed through your system, spending only a little time in your stomach before being converted to blood glucose. Your body reacts to this sugar jolt by releasing a lot of insulin, putting you into a "storage mode" likely to turn a fair amount of the food into fat. Then again, if you're hyperthyroid and seeking to hang on to weight, foods such as potatoes and pasta are healthy, and eating them may help keep you from wasting away.

You can learn how your body will react to a particular food by checking its *glycemic load*, which is a measure of how quickly your blood glucose level will rise after eating it. If you're trying to lose weight, then you'll favor foods with a glycemic load under 10, and ideally under 6. You can get access to lists of foods and their glycemic loads by visiting this book's website at CIGThyroid.com.

> **THYROIDIAN TIP**
>
> If you're hypothyroid, also try to avoid foods with saturated fats (cake, bacon, butter). First, they're calorie intensive. And second, they make your cell membranes resistant to insulin. That means you'll need more insulin than usual to process the same amount of glucose; and since your insulin is already inefficient right now, such foods make a bad situation worse and are likely to turn directly into body fat.

Helping Your Thyroid Work

There are two chemicals that have special importance to your thyroid and that you'll typically take in via food.

The first is *iodine*, which is a fundamental building block for your thyroid's hormone production. Inexpensive and low-calorie food sources for iodine include fresh vegetables grown from iodine-rich soil, fish and shellfish, and the seaweeds nori, wakame, and dulse. To learn more, see Chapter 3.

The second is *selenium*, which plays a role in your body's conversion of T4 to T3 (see Chapter 1). You can solve a selenium shortage by eating a single Brazil nut daily.

In addition, there are two substances you might consider taking for an ailing thyroid. One is the herb ashwagandha, which has virtually no side effects, and can help heal and strengthen glands—including your thyroid.

Finally, if you need to take thyroid medication, seriously consider desiccated thyroid. In addition to such benefits as being the only medication to provide all four thyroid hormones (see Chapter 3), natural thyroid might boost healing. That's because when you consume an animal's gland, the parts of it that aren't digested will be transported by your immune system to the corresponding gland in your body to strengthen it and help rebuild it.

The Least You Need to Know

- Your thyroid is especially vulnerable to unhealthy chemicals, so seek natural foods free of artificial substances and extensive processing.
- Buy organic produce and meats to reduce your intake of pesticides and other toxins.
- If you're hypothyroid, eat foods with a low glycemic load.
- Access lists of foods ranked by pesticide levels, glycemic load, and more at CIGThyroid.com.

Getting That Weight Off

In This Chapter

- Filling up on fiber
- Recording what you eat
- Measuring your RMR and LBM
- Burning fat with T2

If you've been hypothyroid and then prescribed medication, you may have experienced a doctor telling you, "You can go ahead and take that extra weight off now. Good luck." Good luck indeed.

For a fortunate 20 percent of patients, the newly added pounds are magically shed once their metabolism is restored. But if you're like most people, all your stable condition will do is give you the *opportunity* to lose weight. You'll need to actively work at getting your body back in shape. The best advice for doing so has always been "Eat less and exercise more," and we heartily echo that. But this chapter also offers some suggestions that you may not have heard before to help you meet the challenge.

Focusing on Fiber

As explained in Chapter 18, foods that digest slowly and gradually, rather than racing from your stomach to your bloodstream, create less of a sugar jolt and less need for insulin. This puts your body into a calorie burning mode that converts the food into energy (as opposed to a food storage mode that turns it into fat).

One of the best ways to achieve this effect is to choose foods with lots of fiber. Fiber ensures what you eat stays around a while in your stomach and small intestines, making it more likely the food will be burned right away as fuel.

In addition, fiber gives you a feeling of being filled up and satisfied on smaller portions of food—which in turns makes it easier for you to eat less. And fiber makes you want to drink more water, which also fills you up and enables you to get by with less food.

> **THYROIDIAN TIP**
>
> Beyond aiding weight loss, fiber helps your intestines eliminate waste efficiently. The health benefits from this range from flushing out toxins that are bad for your thyroid to preventing constipation (which is a hypothyroid symptom) to guarding against digestive diseases, diabetes, and some cancers. As long as you adjust to it gradually—say, adding 3-4 grams to your diet every few days to avoid bloating—there's really no downside to fiber.

According to nutritional experts, women should eat at least 25 grams of fiber a day and men at least 38 grams a day for overall health. For the purposes of weight loss, it's a good idea to strive for 40 grams a day (for both genders).

Meanwhile, if you're typical, you currently eat less than 15 grams of fiber daily. But that's good news, because it means your diet has lots of room for improvement.

Delicious high-fiber foods include:

- Legumes (navy beans, black beans, pinto beans, adzuki beans, lentils)
- Whole grains (bulgur wheat, oat bran, brown rice)
- Vegetables (spinach, broccoli, eggplant, Brussels sprouts, beets, avocado)
- Fruits (plums, pears, peaches, mangoes, kiwi)
- Berries (blackberries, raspberries, blueberries)
- Nuts (pecans, pistachios, hazelnuts, Brazil nuts)
- Seeds (almonds, flax seeds)

Four high-fiber foods that are especially helpful because they help detoxify you—by flushing unhealthy chemicals and other wastes from your system—are brown rice, beets, flax seeds, and spinach. (Buy organic spinach, though, as the mainstream variety tends to be loaded with pesticides.)

Another great fiber source are adzuki beans (also called aduki beans), which are small reddish beans, typically with a white tip or streak, that are popular in China and Japan. They're packed with magnesium, which plays many vital roles in the body, including aiding thyroid function. Plus, if you're swinging between hypothyroidism and hyperthyroidism, magnesium is a terrific low-impact remedy for stabilizing your heart rate.

In addition, you can get fiber from supplements. One of the most popular is *PGX* (short for *PolyGlycopleX*), which absorbs a great deal of water and so is especially good at filling you up. PGX is inexpensive, readily available from health food stores and online, and can be taken in either capsule or softgel form right before a meal.

Another notable supplement is *inulin*, which is a natural fiber extracted from plants such as Jerusalem artichoke, wild yam, and chicory. Once hard to find, inulin is now readily available in powder form via the commercial product Metamucil Clear & Natural. It's a soluble fiber, meaning it dissolves completely in water; and it's very mildly sweet, so you can add it to smoothies, oatmeal, etc., and barely notice it's there. Just take care to start off gradually to give your body time to adjust to it.

In a nutshell, if counting calories isn't working for you, you may be able to lose weight even more effectively by counting fiber grams. For additional information on this approach, visit website FullPlateDiet.org, which allows you to read an entire fiber-centric diet book online for free.

You can also access detailed lists of high-fiber foods via this book's website at CIGThyroid.com.

Meal Replacements

If you're not great at judging how fattening foods are, you can opt to eat pre-made meals that have a set portion size and set number of calories, such as those sold by Weight Watchers and Healthy Choice.

The previous chapter warned against processed foods, and overall that still holds. But you can eat two meals daily packed with fresh, natural, low-calorie foods, and then substitute the prepared meal for what you'd normally have for dinner. This isn't an ideal way to eat long term; but it can help you lose weight conveniently and sustainably for several months, which may be all you need to return to the body you had before you became hypothyroid.

A spin on this technique is to create the pre-made meal yourself. As long as you're careful about counting calories and fiber—and if you have the patience to prepare your meals in advance—this is an even better approach because it'll teach you the portion control needed to be in charge of your weight.

Yet another spin on this method is to eat only one major protein-based meal daily (typically at dinner). The other two meals can revolve around low-calorie liquids, salads, or even a bowl of very low-sugar cereal and skim milk, to keep you going through the day without slowing down your weight loss.

The trickiest part of this strategy is transitioning back to how you used to eat once you've taken off the extra pounds. But if you're patient and proceed in gradual steps, you can both shed the weight and keep it off.

Food Logging

A large part of the reason we fail to lose weight is that we're relatively oblivious to just how much we eat. Often someone will say, "I don't understand why I'm not losing weight" without realizing that the morning donut and the afternoon milkshake and the post-work beer all add up. Indulging yourself once in a while isn't a problem; what matter are the items you eat and drink regularly as part of your daily routine.

A simple way to address this is to log everything you consume. This ensures that you're paying attention to each morsel that goes into your mouth, and it also makes you think twice when you're about to bite into something that doesn't fit into your meal plan.

Logging food may sound boring, but there are some great online resources to help make the process interactive and fun. Two of them are MyFoodDiary.com and CalorieKing.com. Both websites charge around $12 a month, but in exchange offer databases of over 70,000 foods. These let you quickly look up calorie and nutritional information for virtually any commercial food you can imagine, ranging from basic natural foods to packaged supermarket fare to chain food restaurant offerings; and after you decide to eat the food, the site will automate your recording of it. (For example, MyFoodDiary has a section called "The Fridge" which lets you enter a food you eat frequently with a few mouse clicks.)

Other features of these sites include tracking your calorie, fiber, and sodium intake; an exercise log that calculates your calories burned for over 700 activities; reports that gently encourage you to keep losing (and discourage you from gaining); and online communities to share tips and cheer you on.

Then again, if you do better being cheered by people who are in the same room with you, consider joining face-to-face programs such as Weight Watchers (weightwatchers. com) or Jenny Craig (Jennycraig.com) … which also encourage food logging.

THYROIDIAN TIP

You can buy a measuring scale, complete with a bowl for holding your food, for $20-$30 online. This is very handy if you're working from calorie lists that define food servings in grams or ounces. It also helps you maintain objective portion control—studies have shown we tend to underestimate by an average of 30 percent when gauging food portions by eye alone.

Measuring Your Metabolism and LBM

Your body always has a base level of activity, called your metabolism, that keeps your lungs breathing, your heart beating, and your cells operating to keep you alive. A measure of this base level of activity is your resting metabolic rate, or RMR, which represents the minimum number of calories your body will burn up in 24 hours. Your RMR is responsible for burning up the vast majority of your calories—typically, 65-75 percent. And it's RMR that your thyroid is primarily designed to regulate.

If you're open to spending around $100, you can undergo metabolic testing to learn precisely what your RMR is. This is done via an *indirect calorimetry device* that's available at both health clubs and doctors' offices. It works by having you breathe into a tube for 10-15 minutes while it measures the rate at which you burn oxygen. It then uses this data to very accurately calculate how many calories you burn per day at rest.

You can use this information to figure out how many calories you should eat daily to reach your target weight by a certain date. A good approach is to adopt a diet that comes within 5 percent of your metabolic rate. For example, if you're a 160-pound woman, and metabolic testing has revealed you have an RMR of 1,500 calories, if you consume 1,425-1,575 calories daily and perform light to moderate exercise, you'll lose weight at an ideal rate of 0.5-1.2 pounds per month.

Your initial reaction may be that you'd like to lose weight a lot faster. But setting your caloric intake further below your RMR is a bad strategy. That's because as important as your weight is, even more important is your *lean body mass*, or *LBM*, to body fat ratio. Your lean muscle continually burns calories, and so is a key component of your RMR. If you eat too few calories, though, you won't lose only fat, but also lean muscle tissue. And the less lean muscle you have, the lower your RMR will be. So consuming too little each day is self-defeating.

You *can* slim down quicker. But the way to do it safely is to *exercise*. Performing vigorous exercise at least three times a week increases your lean muscle, which raises your RMR and burns your body fat faster.

To follow your progress in swapping out fat for LBM, you can buy a home bathroom scale that runs a very light current through your body to detect how much fluid you're storing. Such scales aren't 100 percent accurate, but if you get on one the same time every day, and at roughly the same level of hydration, you can get a pretty clear idea of how well you're doing in developing your lean body mass.

One other advantage to losing slowly and steadily is that it's sustainable. If you eat too few calories daily, you'll put your body into a starvation mode that'll make taking off pounds incredibly difficult; and what's likely to follow is binging. Avoid both extremes, as they abuse your body and make subsequent weight loss even more difficult. If your hypothyroidism added 30 or 40 pounds, you shouldn't think of the process of getting them off in terms of weeks or months, but years.

That may seem daunting at first. But if you include exercise as a major component of your weight loss, you may end up with a much better LMB-to-fat ratio than you had before you became hyperthyroid … resulting in your being slimmer and healthier than ever.

 THROAT QUOTE

There's no easy way out. If there were, I would have bought it. And believe me, it would be one of my favorite things!

—Oprah Winfrey

The T2 Factor

If you're on thyroid medication but—despite your best efforts—the weight still isn't coming off, the problem could be a lack of T2. As explained in Chapter 3, most doctors treat hypothyroidism by automatically prescribing Synthroid or its generic version levothyroxine. These are superb medications, but they include only T4. Desiccated thyroid medications, such as Nature-Throid and Armour Thyroid, are the only available sources for T2 aside from the thyroid itself.

Until recently it was assumed T2 did nothing important, and so drug manufacturers had no motivation to create chemical versions of it. Then some researchers decided that if the thyroid makes T2, there's probably a good reason for it; and their studies indicate T2 actually plays a significant role in weight loss.

Specifically, preliminary results show T2 speeds the rate at which the body's cells retrieve and break down fats, which are the first steps in burning your body fat and converting it into energy. T2 also helps offset insulin's effect of putting the body into food storage mode rather than calorie burning mode. And T2 facilitates the conversion of T4 into T3, which raises overall metabolism. Further, studies indicate that T4 seldom converts down to T2.

What we've discussed in this chapter provides a solid foundation for slimming down, and it may be all you need. If you'd care to dig deeper, though, please also read the next chapter on advanced techniques for shedding excess fat.

The Least You Need to Know

- Getting your metabolism back to normal doesn't mean you'll automatically lose the weight you gained while hypothyroid.
- Fiber-rich foods both fill you up and put your body in calorie burning mode.
- Logging everything you eat will lead you to eat less and eat smarter; and online services can make this fun.
- More important than your weight is the ratio of your lean body mass to fat, which means exercise should be a vital component of your weight-loss strategy.
- Try including T2 in your thyroid medications by having your doctor prescribe desiccated thyroid.

Shedding Fat with J. J. Virgin

In This Chapter

- Focusing on excess fat, not pounds
- Being strategic about exercise
- Prioritizing sleep
- Checking for sensitivity to particular foods
- Addressing hormone imbalances

In Chapter 19, we offered basic strategies for losing weight. This chapter digs deeper, providing advanced techniques that will give you a whole new perspective on how to slim down and stay thin.

Unlike the rest of the book, this chapter is the result of an interview Hy had with fitness and nutrition guru J. J. Virgin. J. J. has helped such celebrities as movie stars Ben Stiller, Janeane Garofalo, and Brandon Routh, rock star Gene Simmons, and mega-selling author Jack Canfield, and for two years was the nutrition expert on the *Dr. Phil* show. Suzanne Sommers has said, "Every now and then someone comes along who connects the dots and takes the mystery out of losing weight; J. J. Virgin has done that." In addition to personal coaching, J. J. offers various products through her website www.JJVirgin.com—including her book *Six Weeks to Sleeveless and Sexy.*

Don't Settle for TOFI

Don't focus on being overweight. Aim to stop being "over-fat."

For example, you might be the ideal weight for your height, yet have high body fat and low muscle mass. This is called *TOFI*: thin outside, fat inside. You want to instead be as close to rock-solid as possible.

If you're a woman, you should typically have 18-25 percent body fat; and if you're a man, 10-18 percent fat. (And if you're an athlete, you should be even leaner.)

THYROIDIAN TIP

There are a number of high-end devices for determining body fat. I use a Tanita Segmental scale, because it tells you not only what your body fat is but where it is. Many gyms and doctors keep such a scale in-house and will measure you for an affordable fee.

In order to lose your excess fat and keep it off forever, you must fix what's going on metabolically. Getting your thyroid hormones on track is critical, but you'll usually need to do more than that.

If you're 20 or more pounds over-fat, and you can't manage to lose 1-3 pounds of fat a week despite following a balanced eating plan and exercising, you're what I call "weight loss resistant."

Weight loss resistance can stem from a variety of factors, including poor eating patterns, ineffective exercise, sleep deprivation, food sensitivity, low stomach acid, stress, insulin resistance, and sex hormone imbalances. I'll be addressing all of these issues in this chapter.

Optimize Your Eating Patterns

One of the more unproductive ideas in the diet world is that we need to eat every couple of hours. Eating raises blood sugar, which your cells then burn for energy; but what you actually want them to do is burn off your stored fat for fuel. Frequent eating turns your body into a better sugar burner and a poorer fat burner—the exact opposite of your goal. You should instead settle on a standard three meals a day, with 4-6 hours of no eating between them.

More specifically, you should start each day by taking your thyroid medication (if any), spending 30-60 minutes doing your morning routine, and then eating a substantial breakfast of 500-600 calories.

Breakfast sets your metabolic tone for the day. It's important to start with a slow, steady release of blood sugar. As you then become active, your insulin will drop down to fasting levels, causing your body to use stored fat for fuel.

Studies have shown that someone who eats a breakfast of 500-600 calories is likely to lose as much as 20 pounds more a year than someone who eats a light breakfast of only 300 calories, or skips the meal altogether. You're also more likely to feel better, with improved energy and mental clarity.

You shouldn't go longer than 4-6 hours without eating, though, because that tends to raise stress hormones such as cortisol. So enjoy a light lunch at midday; or if you need to skip lunch, have a mini-meal in the middle of the afternoon.

As for dinner, eat it at least 2-3 hours before going to bed. That's because when you sleep your stomach produces a hormone called *ghrelin* that both makes you hungry and stimulates the secretion of growth hormone. If you've got a full stomach, it'll inhibit the release of ghrelin, and you'll end up with too little hormone for facilitating cell growth and repair. Further, lying down with a full stomach can trigger a washback of stomach acid into your esophagus. Over time this can lead to inflammation, difficulty swallowing, and other problems.

While you should refrain from eating between meals, you should drink lots of water to fill you up. Studies have found that when you're hungry, a glass of water can quickly shut that feeling down. Also good is drinking green tea, which has helpful antioxidants.

CRASH GLANDING

While I encourage green tea between meals, don't drink it *during* meals. Doing so dilutes your stomach acid, making protein digestion less efficient; and you want lots of protein so you can build up your lean body mass.

Drinking Your Meal

Every meal should ideally include protein, fats, non-starchy veggies, and low-sugar carbs. My suggestions on creating balanced meals with these food groups appear in Chapter 21.

If you have problems with portion control, however, or if you're just too busy to prepare all your meals, a simple solution is to replace one meal a day with a protein shake. As long as you're careful to create a drink with the right balance of nutrients and calories, your body won't mind at all.

Whey protein shakes are especially popular. I happen to be sensitive to dairy, so instead use rice pea protein as a base. Whatever your preference, be sure to buy high-quality protein powder. You want it to be easy to digest, and to contain enough protein to make you feel satisfied—25-30 grams if you're a woman, a bit more if you're a man.

I add to that a quarter cup of coconut milk, 1-2 tablespoons of fiber such as flax seed meal, a cup of mixed organic berries, water, and ice. In a couple of minutes, my "meal" is ready to be enjoyed.

This is an easy way to sneak healthy ingredients, such as low-fat protein and fiber, into your diet. Also, it's so convenient that it demolishes any excuse you might have to skip breakfast or lunch because "I don't have time." Even better, studies show that those who replace a meal a day with a shake long-term lose more weight than those who don't … and keep the weight off.

Managing Sweeteners

Another frequent cause of weight loss resistance is too much sugar. Foods and drink with lots of sugar will make your insulin levels skyrocket, bringing your fat burning to an abrupt stop. So when you're making a protein shake or other drink, be sure to limit the sugars to 10 grams total.

Also avoid fructose and fructose-based additives such as agave, which are super-sweet. (Don't be fooled by fructose's low glycemic index.) And be especially wary of eating or drinking something sweet right after working out. Too much sugar will make your body's fat burning efficiency plummet, turning your workout into virtually wasted effort.

> **THYROIDIAN TIP**
>
> It may seem counterintuitive that you can invest 1-2 hours of time and sweat into an exercise session and then derail that work in seconds with a sugary drink. But you need to think of your body as a chemistry lab, not a bank account. Everything has to be working in harmony for your body to burn fat effectively.

Don't use artificial sweeteners, as they put you at risk for too many health problems. I favor natural sugar substitutes such as Xylitol and Stevia. And when actual sugar is required, I use small amounts of evaporated cane juice.

Burst Training

In a society that encourages us to do less and less, I recommend that you push in the other direction and do more. Park your car several blocks from your office so you have to stroll to work, skip the elevator for the stairs, and replace meeting for lunch with a walking date. You can even try wearing a pedometer, which studies have shown motivates us to be more physical. Such movement is good for you, and I want you to think of it as your activity for daily living.

That said, you should *not* view it as an efficient way to slim down. It would take hundreds of hours of casual walking to burn off even 10 pounds.

Along similar lines, endurance-style training such as jogging and cycling for an hour at a time raises stress hormones, and that lowers the effectiveness of T3, testosterone, and growth hormones that help your body build muscle and burn fat. So you may end up putting in a huge amount of time and effort for limited results.

Much more strategic for shedding fat is high-intensity interval training, or *burst training*. For example, instead of walking or jogging for an hour, warm up for a couple minutes, and then sprint as hard as you can for 30-60 seconds. When you're done, walk or jog for 1-3 minutes to recover and allow your heart rate to go back down; and then sprint all out again for another 30-60 seconds.

Don't pace yourself on the sprints; it's better to finish in 30 seconds than in 60, and take double the time to recover. Repeat this pattern for a total of 4-8 minutes. Even this small amount of time invested causes your body to burn fat for a long while afterward.

Burst training isn't exclusive to sprinting. You can do a set by climbing up and down stairs as quickly as you can; pedaling a bike at maximum speed; swimming really fast; jumping rope rapidly; or doing Turkish Get-Ups. (You can find links to videos of me performing the latter, and more, at this book's website CIGThyroid.com.)

Because you don't need a gym or equipment for burst training, you can do it anytime and anywhere that's convenient for you, and mix up the ways you perform sets to keep the exercising fun. The variety also keeps your body challenged.

Once you become used to burst training, you can perform 4-6 sets of 30-60 second bursts, never going beyond a total of 8 minutes. You should do this at least three times a week, preferably on alternate days. (Then again, some of my more athletic clients "burst" every few hours.)

Burst training is time-efficient; a 4-minute workout can achieve the same fat-burning as a 20-minute endurance workout. And while each burst raises your stress hormones, it does so for a very brief period—after which you allow them to come back down. Then you raise them again, and you let them come down again. This effectively trains your sympathetic nervous system to be able to handle higher levels of stress, and recover faster. And fat burning aside, that's an important part of being fit; because true fitness is about being able to keep pushing yourself to do more, but it's also about how quickly you recover.

Another advantage of burst training is the oxygen debt raises your lactic acid, which in turn spurs the production of human growth hormone. So you're causing your body to have an anabolic, or building up, response, not just a breaking down response.

This training will make you stronger in everything you do, and speed your recovery time for all activities. For example, one of my clients was doing endurance-style jogging on a treadmill at 4.5 miles per hour. Her body had become adjusted to this pace, and she'd hit a wall with losing weight. I converted her to burst training, and the fat started sliding off. She was so happy that she stuck to bursts exclusively for 3 months. Then she returned to the treadmill and set it for her normal jog of 4.5 mph; but it suddenly felt like nothing to her. She kept turning up the speed. She finally ended up at 6.4 mph to feel challenged. She couldn't believe the increase in fitness she'd achieved as a side effect of burning fat.

> **THYROIDIAN TIP**
>
> As you get stronger at bursting, don't go longer: go harder. Continue to up the intensity. You'll stay fit as long as you keep pushing to improve.

Strength Training

If you're over the age of 35, your body will start slowly breaking down more muscle and bone than it builds up. That's bad for your overall health, but it's especially a problem when you're trying to shed fat.

First, your muscles are one of the main parts of your body that respond to insulin. If your muscles start decaying, it reduces your body's ability to access stored fat. This is a key cause of weight loss resistance.

Second, muscles require continual energy just to maintain themselves. When you lose muscle mass, your body's energy demands and metabolism decrease, making it that much more difficult to lose weight.

The solution to both problems is *strength training*, which works against the aging process by building your muscles up. Your larger muscles will increase your body's insulin sensitivity, making it easier to access stored fat. And the extra muscles will significantly increase your body's energy needs and so continually burn off more fat. On top of these benefits, you'll look better, feel stronger, and enjoy a healthier life.

> **DEFINITION**
>
> **Strength training** builds up your muscles by increasing their ability to resist force via free weights and other devices. Growing your muscles helps you burn fat by both raising your metabolism and heightening your body's responsiveness to insulin.

You should ideally strengthen all the major muscle groups, which can be organized into four areas:

- **Upper body pushing:** Shoulders, triceps, and chest. Exercises include push-ups, overhead presses, dips, and chest presses (optionally with a big stability ball).

- **Upper body pulling:** Lats (latissimus dorsi), upper back, biceps, shoulders, and back of the shoulders. Exercises include pull-ups, Vancouver rows, one arm rows, and upright rows.

- **Hips and thighs:** Quads, hamstrings, glutes (gluteus maximus), and lower back. Exercises include step-ups, squats, lunges, and plies.

- **Power core:** Lower back (again), abdominals, and obliques. Exercises include crunches, soccer sit ups, and abs on a medicine ball.

Notice that I recommend exercises that work multiple joints simultaneously. For example, do a push-up instead of a simple tricep extension; a pull-up rather than a bicep curl; and a squat in place of a leg extension.

Make use of cables and free weights. And as you become more experienced, vary things up by exercising in progressively imbalanced ways. For example, instead of standing on both feet, try doing free weights while sitting on a ball, or standing on one foot, or lifting a leg up. You want to encourage your body to develop balance and stay stable, because that really activates your core.

Also, do big, full-body movements. It requires a lot more energy, and so has a greater effect.

THYROIDIAN TIP

To get to a range where you're building muscles, do 8-12 repetitions, with a 60-second rest in between sets. The short break gives you some time to recover, but not *too* much. Not totally recovering will recruit more muscle fibers to help on the next set, and that will end up strengthening and building those muscles.

As with any exercise, start out slowly by doing single moderate sets. As you develop strength, though, increase your pace to 2-3 sets, using the heaviest weights you can safely handle in good form. A rule of thumb is that if you can't get to 8 repetitions in a set, you should switch to lighter weights; while if you can easily get past 12 repetitions, you should change up to heavier weights.

I recommend doing strength training at least two times a week, and preferably three times per week for optimal muscle building. Either way, allow for at least a 48-hour rest period in between each session focused on a particular muscle group.

There are a variety of ways you can combine your strength training with your burst training. For example, you can alternate them, doing weights on one day and then bursts the next day. Or you can do burst training followed by working your hips and thighs one day, and then work your upper body and core the next day.

If you can consistently perform both strength training and burst training three times a week, over time you're likely to burn off fat with a speed you never imagined possible.

Getting a Good Night's Sleep

Many people neglect to make sleep a priority, stealing time from it to get in an extra hour or two of work. What they don't realize is that sleep has more of an impact on weight than almost any other lifestyle factor. Studies have shown that even if you're eating right and exercising regularly, failing to get enough sleep puts you at high risk for obesity. There are several reasons for this.

First, your body produces a hormone called ghrelin that gives you an appetite and another called leptin that inhibits appetite. When you don't get enough sleep, your ghrelin levels rise, making you hungry; while your leptin levels fall, making you even hungrier.

Inadequate sleep also lowers your serotonin, and raises your stress hormones and insulin levels. This results in higher blood sugar and the suppression of fat burning.

Further, the effects of greater hunger and lower fat burning are cumulative, getting worse the more nights you skimp on slumber.

To better understand these concepts, imagine yourself waking up without enough sleep. Feeling groggy and weak, you crave carbs and stimulants. You grab a muffin—which is so packed with sugar and fat it's a barely disguised cupcake—and wash it down with a latte. That gives you a sugar rush, and you feel great for a few hours; but then you crash. And your response is to consume even more sugar and caffeine. You end up drinking coffee and caffeinated soda throughout the day. Unfortunately, that creates a brand-new problem, because caffeine remains active in the body for 12 hours.

As you approach nighttime, your adrenaline levels are high when they should be coming down. You respond by drinking a glass of wine; and when that doesn't work, several glasses. You finally become calm enough to fall asleep. But the wine's effects fade after a few hours, waking you in the middle of the night. You get up the next morning feeling unrested … and hungrier than ever for carbs and caffeine.

This is a vicious cycle; and it ends up packing on pounds around your waist. Instead, choose to be good to yourself, and consistently give yourself 7-9 hours of uninter-rupted sleep.

You should ideally go to sleep around the same time every night; fall asleep within 30 minutes of lying down in bed; and wake up around the same time each morning, feeling thoroughly rested.

Dr. Michael Breus recommends creating a routine so consistent that you wake up every morning without the aid of an alarm clock. Instead of setting your alarm for the morning, he suggests you set it to go off at night—to remind you it'll soon be time to go to sleep!

Specifically, he says to set it for an hour before bedtime. That gives you 60 minutes' notice to get ready by powering down. The latter is hugely important. For example, there's been a surge in childhood obesity, and some researchers point to a young person's room having a TV and phone and computer firing up neurons throughout the evening so there's no chance to calm down, lower stress hormones, and sink into a satisfying slumber.

To avoid the same fate, turn off all technology during your power-down hour. Spend the time calmly puttering around with simple chores, or taking a hot bath. Finally, get into bed and start reading a good book … but not a great book! You don't want to get sucked into staying up for a long time, so pick something just entertaining enough to relax you. You should soon feel ready to nod off.

THYROIDIAN TIP

If you aren't satisfied with the quality of your sleep but don't know why, you may find helpful a product called Zeo. Using a headband and software that detect your brain waves, Zeo tracks your stages of sleep and presents detailed data to you in the morning, along with an overall sleep score, so you know what needs improving. To learn more, visit the website MyZeo.com.

Managing Food Sensitivity

A surprising cause of weight loss resistance is sensitivity to particular foods that create havoc as your body tries to deal with their ingestion. This happens more often than you might think; it's estimated 30 percent of us have food sensitivity at some point in our lives.

In some cases the sensitivity is an allergic reaction. A frequent cause is a food making your gut more permeable than it should be and passing through the lining. Your autoimmune system may then respond by identifying the food as an invader and attacking it. This is especially a hazard if you have an autoimmune thyroid disease, as that puts you at greater risk of your immune system finding other targets to assault.

Foods that commonly cause allergic reactions include dairy products (milk, yogurt, cheese), eggs, peanuts, soy products, wheat, seafood, and nuts. Telltale symptoms include sinus issues, throat clearing, moodiness, depression, anxiety, bloating—and, perversely, a craving for the food causing the problem.

A sensitivity can also be a food intolerance. In this case the food doesn't trigger your immune system, but causes a bad reaction because your body has trouble breaking down or digesting it. Common causes of intolerance include the lactose in dairy products; tyrosine, which is in dairy products, soy products, peanuts, almonds, pumpkin seeds, sesame seeds, and lima beans; a variety of preservatives and additives in processed foods; and *gluten*, which is a mix of proteins present in wheat and other grains.

Gluten is an especially frequent culprit, causing such bad reactions as bloating, cramping, inflammation, and problems absorbing nutrients. Gluten is tough to avoid, though, as it hides in thousands of products, including:

- Bread and bread crumbs
- Pasta and semolina
- Bulgar wheat, couscous, and farina
- Cookies, muffins, scones, cake, pies
- Cereals with wheat, barley, or rye
- Sausages and luncheon meats (often contain bread)
- Blue cheeses (often contain bread)

- Seitan (is pure wheat gluten)
- Most packaged foods (often contain bread)

You can find a more complete list at this book's website, CIGThyroid.com.

If you have any reason to suspect a sensitivity to certain foods, the best thing to do is cut them completely out of your diet for a full month and see if you notice any changes in your health and/or your fat loss. If you don't, you can eliminate this as a potential issue.

If you *do* have a sensitivity, though, you may start intensely craving the food causing your problems. You may also feel a lot worse for the first few days, experiencing bloating, diarrhea, headaches, and so on. Once your body adjusts, however, such uncomfortable feelings will go away; plus you may well drop around five pounds.

After a month has gone by, you can slowly and cautiously reintroduce one particular food at a time to see whether symptoms reappear. If they do, you'll know that you need to avoid that food (or the group of foods it represents). But sometimes you can rotate a "problem" food back into your diet so long as you take care to eat it only once in a while.

Managing Low Stomach Acid

As you become older, your stomach acid may decrease. This can also happen as a result of food sensitivity, or from stress. When this occurs, it impairs digestion, and especially protein digestion, making you feel full but not satisfied. The loss of protein will reduce your body's ability to grow new hormones, muscles, bones, skin, hair, nails, and so on.

An even more serious issue for weight loss is that your stomach acid is normally the first line of defense for killing invaders that come in through food. When your stomach acid is low, it creates an environment that allows for bacterial overgrowth in the small intestine; and this can lead to your body extracting more calories from the foods you eat and storing them as fat.

One of my clients had exactly this problem. Within a few months of our figuring out what was going on and addressing it, she lost *40 pounds*. So gut bacterial overgrowth can have a profound effect on your weight.

This is why I tell clients to not take probiotics blindly. While the microorganisms in probiotics are normally beneficial, they can add to a bacterial problem when your stomach acid is low. A telltale sign for this issue is becoming bloated as the day goes on, whether you eat or not. If you notice this happening, have your doctor run a urine organic acid test that looks for gut *dysbiosis* (meaning "out of balance").

If you test positive, you can typically eliminate the overgrowth via a round of antibacterial herbs, such as enteric-coated peppermint oil, garlic, ginger, grapefruit seed extract, olive leaf extract, bergerine, or echinacea. If necessary, you can also take prescription antibiotics.

Of course, that still leaves you with low stomach acid. Generally the best way to address this is with *betaine HCl*, which raises stomach acid. Do this cautiously, though, by taking one pill with a meal that includes protein and seeing how it makes you feel. If that goes well, increase the dosage to two pills per meal. Gradually keep increasing the number of pills (up to a maximum of eight) over the course of a number of meals until you feel the mildest little burn, and then reduce the dosage by one pill. Most people end up taking 3-6 pills per meal initially, and over time decrease that to 2-4 per meal.

Then again, if you prefer food to a pill, try regularly eating pineapple or papaya, which have acid-raising properties.

CRASH GLANDING

If you have a history of ulcers, gastritis, or gastrointestinal symptoms such as heartburn, you typically should *not* take an acid-raising medication such as betaine HCl. Instead, consult with your doctor about the best course of treatment.

Managing Stress

When you suffer from stress, an array of bad things happen. The stress hormone cortisol rises, which leads to higher blood sugar and reduced fat burning. At the same time, it lowers serotonin and leptin levels, making you hungrier. This awful combination is a formula for adding fat around your waist.

Stress also lowers the sex hormones DHEA and testosterone, hampering your ability to build up muscle.

In addition, stress lowers your stomach acid, which makes it more difficult for your body to digest protein and use the protein to create muscles.

Further, if the stress continues over a long period, your adrenal glands will eventually reverse gears and produce too *little* cortisol. At that point you'll be relying on adrenaline for energy, or just have very little energy. If you then try to address your weight gain by cutting calories and/or engaging in endurance-style training, you may strain your adrenal glands to the point of doing lasting damage.

Once things get to this point, you may need to spend several months healing your body by eliminating stress, getting consistent and uninterrupted sleep, eating balanced meals, and performing burst training in moderation via 4-minute sessions. (For ways to specifically heal your adrenal glands, see Chapter 14.)

It's not always possible to eliminate the source of your stress. However, you can often change your reaction to it, which will be just as effective in making your stress disappear. For more ideas on how to cut stress from your life—both for weight loss and overall health—see Chapter 22.

Managing Insulin Resistance

If your diet consists mostly of carbs and fructose, you're pushing your blood sugar levels through the roof. Your pancreas reacts by pumping out insulin to lower your blood sugar. That works for a while. Over time, however, the cell receptors designed to respond to insulin become overloaded by the barrage, and desensitized. This makes your body partially resistant to insulin—and forces your pancreas to pump out even more insulin to achieve the effects it used to. This vicious cycle can make your cells increasingly insulin resistant.

At the same time, high levels of insulin effectively lock the doors to your fat cells, making it very hard for your body to burn stored fat for fuel. It also creates inflammation, which is an independent risk factor for weight loss resistance. And fat aside, excessive insulin raises your risk for high blood pressure, heart attacks, and other major diseases.

Fortunately, you can repair your body by doing a lot of the things that have already been recommended in this chapter:

- **Eat balanced meals with low sugar and lots of fiber.** This will lower your blood sugar, and so reduce insulin production.

- **Eliminate stress.** This will also lower blood sugar.

- **Get 7-9 hours of uninterrupted sleep every night.** Sleep deprivation is a major contributor to insulin resistance.

- **Do strength training.** It's a great way to improve insulin sensitivity.

In addition, try any or all of the following:

- Take fish oil pills, which reduce inflammation and help resensitize your cells' insulin receptors.

- Take conjugated linoleic acid (CLA) and/or lipoic acid, which also help resensitize your cells' insulin receptors.

- Take chromium, vanadium, magnesium, and zinc, which help manage blood sugar.

- Determine your vitamin D levels with a test called *25-hydroxyvitamin D*, and then take supplements (or spend more time in the sun) to get your vitamin D to 60-80 mgs per mL, which studies have shown combats insulin resistance.

THYROIDIAN TIP

Often occurring simultaneously with insulin resistance is resistance to leptin, a hormone that suppresses appetite. This creates a nightmare scenario of getting hungrier, and eating more, as your ability to burn fat decreases. Fortunately, most of the remedies just described for insulin resistance will cure leptin resistance as well.

Managing Sex Hormones

Whether you're a man or woman, testosterone is critical to weight loss, because it helps you burn fat and build muscle. Unfortunately, your testosterone decreases as you get older. This means as you move past middle age, you're likely to start developing belly fat unless you do something about it.

If you're a woman, you have the additional burden of your cortisol levels rising as you approach menopause, putting you at risk for all the problems discussed in the previous section. Plus your estrogen and progesterone will become unbalanced, which often leads to increased fat retention.

As you know if you have thyroid disease, it's really hard to fight against your hormones. But that doesn't mean you have to give in to your body when it's telling you to lose muscle and store fat. Instead, have a hormone specialist get you on bioidentical hormone replacement therapy. In other words, make testosterone and other sex hormones work for you instead of against you.

If you continue to take great care of your body, your 50s and 60s can be the best years of your life.

The Least You Need to Know

- More important than your weight is your ratio of fat to lean body mass.
- The most effective exercises for burning off fat are burst training and strength training.
- One of the most important things you can do to keep burning fat is consistently get a good night's sleep.
- If you can't lose weight while craving a particular food, avoid that food for a month to see whether you're sensitive to it.
- If you become bloated whether you eat or not, get tested for gut bacterial overgrowth.

Planning Meals

A lot of people have the notion that healthy meals take too long to prepare, aren't as tasty as processed food, and are too expensive.

None of those things are true. Preparation time is essentially the same. It's just a matter of getting past the learning curve of working with different ingredients. And fresh, natural food is considerably more delicious than processed. All that's required is giving up the unhealthy stimulation provided by additives such as MSG and corn syrup. As for expense, fresh produce is typically cheaper than processed foods. You can even buy organic at reasonable prices if you're a smart shopper who supports local farms.

This chapter offers suggestions on how to create meals that are healthy for your thyroid and your whole body, and will help you lose weight. The meals are broken down into three basic components: fruits and vegetables, proteins, and carbohydrates.

THROAT QUOTE

Nearly everyone wants at least one outstanding meal a day.

—Duncan Hines

Fruits and Vegetables

Produce should ideally take up half the volume of a meal. We suggest buying your fruits and vegetables as fresh as possible, which ensures they contain lots of antioxidants—special molecules that help maintain your overall health. An added benefit is they're more delicious when recently picked. If possible, buy organic to obtain a denser level of nutrients, better flavor, and fewer toxins. Alternatively, mix mainstream and organic produce strategically.

If you don't have time to shop for all fresh veggies, the next best thing is frozen vegetables, which are typically preserved at the peak of their freshness. Just take care to buy ones that are minimally processed and have nothing added to them.

Strive to buy as many different colors of produce as you can. The variety of a fruits-and-veggies "rainbow" helps ensure you're getting all the nutrients your body needs.

The USDA has set the serving size of produce to be a cup raw (about the size of your fist) or half a cup cooked. Studies indicate 10 such servings a day of fruits and vegetables drastically reduces the risk of disease, including heart problems, stroke, and most cancers.

Like your parents have always said, eat your vegetables. They really are good for you.

THYROIDIAN TIP

If a fruit is starting to lose its freshness but you aren't ready to eat it, consider freezing it for later use in a smoothie. This is an especially useful strategy for bananas; simply peel them, toss them in a sealable plastic bag, and then store them in your freezer until you need a healthy sweetener for a blended drink.

Proteins

Protein is a vital component of any healthy diet. Your body uses protein to make and transport your hormones (including your thyroid's T4, T3, and T2). It also uses protein to grow and repair your cells.

A protein should comprise about a quarter of the volume of a meal. The serving size should typically be around the size of a deck of cards.

As with produce, organic is the best choice. You can often find bargains via local family farms and ranches (see Chapter 18). But whether organic or mainstream, if it's an animal protein, it should be as low in fat as possible. The toxins animals eat are stored in their fat, and you don't want these poisons passed along to you. So buy lean, cut away fat, remove skin, and favor white meat over dark.

Great protein sources include fish, shellfish, white meat poultry, and lean red meat such as buffalo and ostrich (preferably grass fed). Also great are eggs, cottage cheese, tofu, tempeh, and seitan. Regarding the last three items: even if you're not a vegetarian, it's wise to have a large number of animal-free meals as part of your menu plan for variety, and to lessen the load on your system from any toxins you might be consuming when going up the food chain.

In fact, a lifestyle gaining popularity is that of the *flexitarian*. This is someone who mostly eats vegetarian dishes but eats meat as well. It's a way of minimizing toxins while still having access to the complete protein meat provides.

Carbohydrates

A carbohydrate-based food should fill up the remaining quarter of your meal. As suggested in Chapter 19, focus on carbs with a lot of fiber. They'll take longer to enter your bloodstream, making it more likely they'll be burned as fuel rather than stored as fat. And the fiber will both fill you up (so you feel satisfied with less food) and enhance your overall health.

If you're trying to lose weight, you should aim for 40 grams of fiber a day, which means any meal should ideally contain 10-15 grams. Along the same lines, keep sugar low, because it's likely to kick your body into food storage mode and pack on pounds. A good goal is consuming under 40 grams of sugar a day, which translates to under 15 grams per meal. That means staying away from soda, sauces, fruit juices (stick to fresh fruit), and even sugary yogurts.

As with all foods, vary your choices. If you have brown rice one night, have bulgur wheat the next, and couscous after that. This ensures you're not missing any nutrients; and it makes meals livelier.

THYROIDIAN TIP

Cook quicker and easier using modern tools. For example, bread machines allow you to choose your own ingredients—which can include organic flour, and as much fiber as you like—and can be set to turn on while you're at work so you can come home to fresh-baked bread. And a rice cooker lets you just pour in the grains, along with water or chicken broth, and have brown rice come out perfect every time. The cooker also does a great job with other grains, such as steel-cut oats, amaranth, and quinoa.

Balancing Meals with J. J. Virgin

In case your main interest is slimming down, we're also sharing the advice of J. J. Virgin, a renowned fitness and nutrition guru (see Chapter 20).

I recommend every meal include protein, healthy fat, non-starchy veggies, and a high-fiber carb. The amount of protein you eat should be based on your lean body mass (LBM), using a formula of 0.7-1 gram of protein per pound.

If your current LBM is far from the LBM you want to have, though, then add the two numbers and divide by two, and use that average for the formula. (And remember to keep adjusting the average as you get closer to your goal.)

Once you determine your ideal amount of protein, spread it across your three daily meals. In addition to protein's health benefits, it tends to suppress the production of the hunger hormone ghrelin, helping you to feel sated and eat less.

As for fat, I recommend 1-3 servings at every meal. Fat triggers the release of a chemical in the small intestine called *cholecystokinin* that tells your brain you're full. When you're not hungry, you're not as likely to overeat.

You should stick to healthy fat, though: raw nuts and seeds, extra virgin olive oil, coconut oil, coconut milk, avocados, and olives. Ideal are omega-3 and monounsaturated fat, which are anti-inflammatories that help protect you against disease. They also make your cell membranes more fluid and better able to communicate with your hormones.

CRASH GLANDING

You should *not* include peanuts on your list of "healthy fat" nuts. Despite their name, peanuts are legumes; and they're also inflammatories.

The foods I want to see most on your plate are non-starchy vegetables. Every day you should ideally eat 5-10 servings. This will give you plant nutrients, called phytonutrients; and fiber, which (like protein) keeps ghrelin suppressed so you're not hungry. Fiber also speeds food through your intestine, lowers bad cholesterol and raises the good kind … and helps you develop buttocks you can be proud of.

Finally, you should eat 1 or 2 servings of a high-fiber starchy carb and low-sugar fruit. Examples of these includes brown rice, sweet potatoes, black beans, and lentils; and berries, apples, peaches, and plums.

So a typical meal could be some salmon (protein), a cup of lentil soup (high fiber carbs), and some spinach and mushrooms (veggies) sautéed at low heat in extra virgin olive oil (healthy fat).

Eating Out

In our fast-paced world, it's become common to obtain a large percentage of our calories by eating out. Restaurants are convenient, but they typically aren't focused on your health. Their goal is to serve flavor enhancers and calorie-intense foods delivering an addictive sugar jolt that keeps customers coming back. You can get a nourishing and moderate-calorie meal at a restaurant, but it requires some smart planning.

First, be prepared to be picky about condiments. Figure on skipping the sour cream, mayonnaise, butter, syrups, sauces, and oils. Instead, focus on low-fat and low-calorie condiments such as mustard, ketchup, salsa, vinegar, and chutney. Along the same lines, always get dressing, gravy, etc., on the side. You can then have precisely as much or little as you want. For example, instead of pouring dressing on your salad, dip your fork in the dressing and then dig into the salad. You'll get the flavor of the dressing, but with way fewer calories.

And speaking of salads, be sure to have one with your meal. If a salad isn't included with your entrée, order it as a side dish or as a substitute for something unhealthy such as oil-soaked french fries.

Also be aware that a restaurant will typically serve you twice as many calories as you really should consume in one meal. If you're eating with a group, consider ordering fewer entrées than the number of people in your party and sharing the food among yourselves communally. That way you can collectively eat everything on the plates without anyone feeling stuffed.

Alternatively, if you're eating alone, ask for a take-out container at the same time you're ordering, and when your meal arrives put half of the food in the container. This ensures you don't overload your system with calories and trigger your body's food storage mode; plus it provides you with a delicious meal of leftovers for the next day.

THROAT QUOTE

The most remarkable thing about my mother is that for 30 years she served the family nothing but leftovers. The original meal has never been found.

—Calvin Trillin

Embracing Goitrogens

You may have heard that cruciferous vegetables—such as broccoli, cauliflower, cabbage, Brussels sprouts, and kale—are bad for your thyroid. They *do* contain indole-3-carbinol, which can inhibit your thyroid's ability to absorb iodine. As a result, they're sometimes called goitrogens because when consumed in large quantities they have the ability to spur hypothyroidism, which in turn can lead to goiters. But if you eat normal daily amounts of these veggies—up to two cups (100 grams) raw or five cups cooked—you needn't worry about this. Cruciferous vegetables are among the healthiest foods on the planet, so don't deprive yourself of them.

You may have heard similar negative things about soy products, which are also goitrogens. That's because soy contains isoflavones, which can interfere with iodine being digested properly and reaching your thyroid. However, you'd have to eat an awful lot of soy for this to become an issue. As long as your daily consumption doesn't go above two servings—100 grams of soy food or six ounces of soy milk—don't worry about this, either.

The Least You Need to Know

- An ideal meal in volume should be half fruits and vegetables, a quarter protein, and a quarter carbohydrates.
- Buy a rainbow of produce to get a variety of nutrients, and eat produce fresh to maximize antioxidants.

- Minimize your consumption of toxins from meat by buying lean, cutting away fat, and eating more vegetarian meals.

- Plan on eating only half of a calorie-intense restaurant meal and taking the rest home for the next day.

- Enjoy cruciferous vegetables and soy products, which will do your thyroid no harm when eaten in moderation.

Living Better

In This Chapter

- Avoiding mercury, perchlorate, and fluoride
- Eliminating household toxins
- Getting stress out of your life
- Appreciating exercise

Chapter 18 described toxins in processed foods, produce, and meat that have the potential to disrupt your thyroid. Unfortunately, there are also other sources of dangerous chemicals you need to be aware of. In this chapter we describe some of the most notable environmental threats to your thyroid, and ways you can avoid them.

In addition, we discuss how to mitigate the intangible toxin stress, which can wear down your thyroid as well as the rest of your body.

Finally, we point out some of the immense benefits of exercise.

We hope the suggestions that follow help you enjoy a longer, healthier, and happier life.

Thyroid Threats

As explained in Chapter 1, your thyroid is designed to suck every bit of iodine out of your bloodstream and store it until needed. The problem is your thyroid will also draw in artificial chemicals that make their way into your bloodstream and that your body was never designed to handle.

While this can happen with a number of chemicals, there are certain ones to which your thyroid is especially vulnerable because their composition is very similar to that of iodine. Your thyroid will absorb every molecule of these it can find and permanently store them. As they accumulate, they can interfere with your thyroid's functioning by displacing iodine, doing direct physical damage to your thyroid, and/ or attracting the attention of your immune system, leading to an autoimmune disease such as Hashimoto's or Graves'.

The three substances most likely to threaten your thyroid because of their chemical resemblance to iodine are mercury, perchlorate, and fluoride.

Mercury

Mercury is a dangerous poison found in minute amounts in thousands of processed foods. Mercury is also present in fish. You don't want to avoid eating seafood, because most of it is good for you. However, it's wise to refrain from consuming fish likely to have the highest levels of mercury—which are swordfish, thresher sharks, and marlin.

Also worrisome is tuna. While its mercury levels aren't as high as those of the somewhat exotic fish just mentioned, tuna is eaten so frequently that its mercury can accumulate at an alarming rate. And counterintuitively, it's the highest-quality tuna that poses the greatest risk. That's because top-grade tuna comes from larger, older fish, and they're the ones that have lived long enough to build up the most mercury in their bodies. So you're at lowest risk eating flaked "light" tuna, at moderate risk with albacore, at significant risk with the "tuna steak" grade … and you probably shouldn't even think about consuming sushi-grade tuna beyond rare occasions.

> **THYROIDIAN TIP**
>
> You can find out how much tuna is safe for you to eat based on your gender and weight by visiting a tuna calculator provided by the Environmental Working Group at EWG.org/tunacalculator.

If you suspect you're suffering from mercury poisoning, talk to your doctor about getting tested for it. The process involves taking a dose of mercury chelating medicine—which removes heavy metals from your body—and then providing your urine. By measuring the amount of mercury that comes out of your body, a lab can estimate how much mercury is stored in your thyroid.

Perchlorate

Another chemical similar enough to iodine to fool your thyroid is perchlorate. While not as poisonous as mercury, perchlorate is a byproduct of rocket fuel production, so it's hardly people friendly. Studies have found even low levels of perchlorate can interfere with the thyroid's ability to absorb iodine, leading to hypothyroidism.

Perchlorate has been found in the water supplies of over 35 U.S. states. You can learn if it's been detected in your local water supply by visiting the U.S. Environmental Protection Agency's site at EPA.gov/safewater/dwinfo. If it has, the simplest way to avoid perchlorate is to drink bottled water from a source that either has no perchlorate or filters out such impurities.

THYROIDIAN TIP

Another way to avoid perchlorate is to install a special filter in your home that purifies your tap water. Most conventional filters (Brita, PUR) won't do the job in this case, but a reverse osmosis system designed to trap perchlorate will. This can cost as little as $150, plus $20-$30 filter changes 1 or 2 times per year.

Fluoride

In contrast to toxins, fluoride is so relatively safe that many communities have put it in their water supply to fight tooth decay. At the same time, its ubiquitousness has led experts to wonder if fluoride is partly to blame for the current hypothyroidism epidemic.

Like mercury and perchlorate, fluoride is chemically similar to iodine. The more fluoride your thyroid absorbs, the less room there is for iodine; and the more likely it is that the fluoride will block iodine from your thyroid's hormone construction sites. The result is a substantial reduction in thyroid hormones.

Fluoride is so effective at reducing T4 and T3 production that it's used as a treatment for hyperthyroidism (see Chapter 12). If you're on the verge of being hypothyroid, though, fluoride is likely to push you over the edge. And if you're already hypothyroid, fluoride can make your condition even worse.

If fluoride is in your local water supply, you can avoid it by drinking bottled water; or, as mentioned for perchlorate, by installing a reverse osmosis filter for your tap water.

Cutting Down on Chemicals

While mercury, perchlorate, and fluoride are the best-known threats to your thyroid, they're far from the only ones. Any modern artificial chemical, or combination of chemicals, could have an unexpectedly adverse affect. Your best defense is to avoid as many of them as possible.

For example, a 2010 study found people with high levels of the chemical *perfluorooctanoic acid*, or *PFOA*, are twice as likely to have thyroid disease. PFOA is used in nonstick Teflon cookware, microwave popcorn bags, stain-resistant carpet and fabric coatings, and certain cleansers.

Most of these are products you can live without. For example, you can use enamel-coated cast iron pans instead of Teflon; and you can microwave air-pop popcorn using brown paper lunch bags.

As for cleansers, you should ideally buy organic versions that contain no harmful chemicals. These include Dr. Bronner's Sal Suds, Natural Soap Formula's KD Gold, and a line of green products from Seventh Generation. (For a list of websites offering these products, and more, visit this book's site at CIGThyroid.com.)

You can also use old-fashioned but still effective solutions, such as white vinegar and water on newspapers for cleaning windows, weakly brewed black tea for mirrors, lemon juice or vinegar for most stains, club soda for carpet stains, and cornmeal for spills. (For further details and suggestions, visit CIGThyroid.com.)

Similarly, you should choose organic products in place of:

- Artificial pesticides, especially when spraying inside your house (for instance, try boric acid, which is nontoxic).

- Chemical-based cosmetics and body care products.

- Insecticide- and herbicide-saturated wines and beers.

Most chemical engineers are never trained in toxicology, which means they invent new chemicals without deep knowledge of the potential effects on people. This has caused untold misery. In response, a green, organic movement has developed that allows you to live a safer, more natural, and healthier life. Don't hesitate to join it.

Shrinking Stress

Stress can have just as negative an impact on you as toxins. A common result of our fast-paced lives, stress triggers an adrenaline rush that raises your heart rate, makes your breath quicker, and moves your blood away from your organs toward your skeletal muscles, readying you to respond by either fighting or fleeing.

This worked great when our ancestors regularly faced off against tigers and rival tribes. However, it's not as helpful when you're being criticized by your boss or stuck in a traffic jam.

Stress impairs your digestive system, your immune system, and your body's ability to repair itself. If sustained for a long time, it'll wear you down and make you sick. Some experts believe stress is one of the reasons serious diseases—including thyroid disease—are on the rise.

You don't have to helplessly suffer, though. There are a number of things you can try to reduce stress:

- **Avoid the person stressing you out.** If it's a friend or colleague, be polite but firm. If it's your manager and the stress is unending, consider finding another job.

- **Avoid the situation stressing you out.** For example, if standing in line is aggravating, get your chores done during non-peak hours or hire someone to do them for you.

- **Say "no."** If you really don't want to do something, then don't.

- **Talk it out.** If it's not possible to say "no," then tactfully express your frustration. Maybe a compromise can be reached.

- **Focus on what fulfills you.** If you love spending time with your family, figure out ways to do more of that. If you have a book burning inside you, carve out an hour every morning or evening to work on it—with no excuses.

- **Adjust your perspective.** Sometimes if you decide to not let something bother you, it won't.

- **Do something calming.** Meditation, yoga, visualization, gardening, listening to music … whatever relaxes you is good.

- **Breathe.** Breathe in through your nose for seven seconds, and then breathe out through your mouth for seven seconds. This can be remarkably effective.

- **Laugh.** Go to a live comedy show, see a funny film, or spend some time with four-year-olds—whatever it takes.

- **Sleep.** There are few things in life as healing as enough sleep. If you've been depriving yourself, revise your priorities to ensure a full eight hours each night.

- **Cut out stimulants.** If you're drinking a lot of coffee or soda, switch to a beverage without caffeine.

- **Help others.** Caring for other people in need—or even pets—may make you feel differently about your own troubles.

- **Be physical.** Take a walk in the park ... or better yet, a jog. Lift weights. Exercise. Any physical activity may help satisfy your body's "fight or flight" response.

Stress can be as debilitating as any disease. Don't let it damage your quality of life.

Embracing Exercise

It's been said that if exercise was a pill, every doctor would prescribe it. Exercise is a great antidote for stress. It can also help cure depression, anxiety, and many other ills.

Exercise strengthens every part of your body, ranging from your immune system to your hair and skin to your libido to your mind. In the past it was thought exercise could wear out joints. We now know that even the worst arthritis improves over time with exercise. Exercise can also increase energy and enthusiasm, and improve the quality of your sleep. Exercise lowers your risks for cancer, heart disease, diabetes, Alzheimer's, and stroke.

And as Chapter 20 explains, strategic exercises such as burst training and strength training are invaluable tools for weight loss.

If you're perpetually tired and are chalking it up to old age, it may be that you're just not getting enough exercise. A 2010 study found that regular exercise can delay aging by as much as *12 years.*

If you haven't exercised for a while, go slow. Do a little, give yourself a day or two to recover, and then do a little more. The rest periods will provide your body the time it needs to adapt ... and to build itself up for a healthier and happier new you.

The Least You Need to Know

- Eat seafood 1 or 2 times a week, but reduce or eliminate fish that are known for containing a lot of mercury.

- If your local water supply has perchlorate and/or fluoride, drink bottled or purified water.

- Eliminate stress by ending the cause of it, avoiding the source of it, or changing your response to it.

- Make exercise an integral part of your life. There's nothing better you can do for your health.

Glossary

AACE   American Association of Clinical Endocrinologists (aace.com).

ACTH   Adrenocorticotropic hormone or corticotropin, which is made by your pituitary glands to regulate the hormone production of your adrenal glands.

Addison's disease   A physical problem with your adrenal glands (such as a genetic defect) or an autoimmune disorder in which they're being attacked by antibodies, that causes them to underperform. Also called adrenal insufficiency.

adenoma   A small non-cancerous growth.

adenosine triphosphate   See *ATP*.

adrenal glands   Two small triangle-shaped lumps of tissue residing over your kidneys that produce cortisol, which (among other things) helps convert T4 into T3, and allows T3 to enter cell membranes and access mitochondria.

adrenaline   A hormone produced by your adrenal glands in response to dangerous or unexpected situations. Adrenaline increases your heart rate, expands your blood vessels and air passages, and makes other subtle changes that help you react instantly by either battling or running (fight or flight).

adrenocorticotropic hormone   See *ACTH*.

alpha-lipoic acid   See *lipoic acid*.

antibodies   Proteins used by your immune system to attack foreign invaders, such as bacteria and viruses. When your immune system mistakes your thyroid as a threat, it may attack those cells with thyroid peroxidase antibodies (TPO) and/or thyroglobulin antibodies (Tg), resulting in Hashimoto's disease; or with thyroid stimulating immunoglobulin antibodies (TSI), resulting in Graves' disease.

antithyroid medications   Drugs such as Tapazole/methimazole and propylthiouracil (PTU) that manage hyperthyroidism by interfering with your thyroid's ability to make its hormones.

Armour Thyroid   Medication made from desiccated pig thyroid that contains all four thyroid hormones: T4, T3, T2, and T1. Manufactured by Forest Laboratories (ArmourThyroid.com and FRX.com).

ashwagandha   Traditional Ayurvedic herb (Latin name *withania somnifera*) that can help heal and strengthen glands, including the thyroid and adrenal glands. Ashwagandha is Sanskrit for "smells like a horse," but in its commercial form its odor is typically neither strong nor unpleasant, and it has virtually no side effects.

atenolol   A beta blocker that's effective at slowing a rapid heartbeat caused by hyperthyroidism.

ATP   Adenosine triphosphate, the energy created from the conversion of glucose by the mitochondria in your cells.

autoimmune disease   A condition in which your immune system mistakenly attacks an area of your body. Over 80 percent of thyroid disease cases are caused by the autoimmune diseases Hashimoto's (hypothyroidism) and Graves' (hyperthyroidism), both of which attack your thyroid with antibodies.

basal temperature test   An old-fashioned test used to identify hypothyroidism via body temperature. It's been made obsolete by modern lab tests, which are much more reliable and precise.

benzodiazepines   Medications that are effective at managing anxiety caused by hyperthyroidism, including Valium, Xanax, Dalmane, and Tranxene.

beta blocker   A medication that blocks the effects of adrenaline, making your heart beat more slowly and with less force. It also helps reduce your blood pressure and improve your blood's circulation. The best beta blockers for hyperthyroidism include atenolol and propranolol.

betaine HCl   Medication used to combat *low stomach acid*. The typical dosage is 2-4 pills at every meal that includes protein, but can vary for each person. You typically shouldn't use an acid-raising medication such as betaine HCl if you have a history of ulcers, gastritis, or gastrointestinal symptoms such as heartburn. Consult your doctor for details.

biopsy   See *fine needle aspiration biopsy* and *coarse needle biopsy*.

block-and-replace therapy   A technique for managing hyperthyroidism in which your doctor blocks the disease with antithyroid medication while simultaneously replacing any lack of hormones with thyroid medication.

Brazil nut   Your best source of selenium. Eat just one a day; more risks an eventual selenium overdose.

bromocriptine   A medication used to slow the growth of, and often shrink, an adenoma on the pituitary gland.

burst training   Also called high-intensity interval training, this workout method involves exerting yourself as hard as you can (by sprinting, swimming, etc.) for 30-60 seconds, resting for 1-3 minutes, and then exerting yourself all-out again. Burst training typically burns fat much more efficiently than conventional exercise such as walking or jogging. Burst training works best when combined with *strength training*.

cancer   See *thyroid cancer*.

carnitine   See *L-carnitine*.

cholecystokinin   A hormone that stimulates the digestion of fat and suppresses hunger. One reason to eat a moderate amount of healthy fat every meal is to produce this hormone, which effectively tells your brain that you're full and so makes you less likely to overeat.

coarse needle biopsy   A procedure for a potentially cancerous nodule three quarters of an inch or larger; it employs a needle to extract tissue samples for examination in a lab. See also *fine needle aspiration biopsy*.

cold nodule   See *thyroid nodule*.

compounded thyroid medication   Thyroid medication prepared by a compounding pharmacy instead of a drug manufacturer (which has greater quality assurance and post-production analysis). It's normally fine to use a compounding pharmacy, but thyroid hormones are so minute that the risk of a mistake being made outweighs any convenience gained by compounding.

comprehensive metabolic panel (CMP)   A very common test that identifies the levels of a variety of critical chemicals in your bloodstream, including calcium (which is useful if you suspect a problem with your parathyroid glands). Also called a chemistry panel, chemistry screen, and SMAC test.

conjugated linoleic acid (CLA)   A natural dietary supplement that can help combat *insulin resistance* by re-sensitizing insulin cell receptors. See also *lipoic acid*.

corticotropin   See *ACTH*.

cortisol   A critical hormone produced by your adrenal glands. Its many functions include regulating your blood's glucose levels, controlling your blood pressure, healing inflammation, helping convert T4 into T3, and allowing T3 to enter cell membranes and access mitochondria.

cortisol challenge test   A test in which you're given a small dose of ACTH to see how much cortisol your adrenal glands produce in response, which provides precise information on your adrenals' health. See also *salivary cortisol testing*.

Cushing's syndrome   A condition in which weight gain, weakened immunity, thinning skin and hair, and other problems are caused by too much cortisol. See also *pheochromocytoma*.

Cytomel   Thyroid medication that's a synthetic version of T3, manufactured by King Pharmaceuticals (KingPharm.com). The generic version is liothyronine.

cytopathologist   A doctor who's an expert at analyzing cells extracted via a biopsy.

deiodinase type 1   The enzyme your body uses to strip off an iodine atom from a thyroid hormone molecule and convert it into a different hormone—most notably, turning T4 into T3. See also *selenium*.

desiccated thyroid   Medication made from desiccated pig thyroid that contains all four thyroid hormones: T4, T3, T2, and T1. Also called glandular thyroid, natural desiccated thyroid, or NDT. Brand name versions of this medication include Armour Thyroid, Nature-Throid, and WesThroid.

desiccated thyroid powder   The raw material used to make desiccated thyroid, manufactured by American Laboratories (AmericanLaboratories.com).

do-iodothyronine   See *T2*.

dulse   A seaweed that's an excellent source of iodine.

endocrine system   A group of glands that secrete hormones regulating how your body functions. The glands include the thyroid, parathyroids, pancreas, ovaries, testes, adrenals, pineal, pituitary, and hypothalamus.

endocrinologist   A doctor who specializes in disorders of the glands of the endocrine system and their hormones.

ENT   Ear, nose, and throat surgeon, which is typically the doctor needed for thyroid cancer.

eye disease   See *hyperthyroid eye disease*.

fine needle aspiration biopsy   A procedure that employs a very thin needle to extract tissue samples from any potentially cancerous nodules on your thyroid for examination in a lab. See also *coarse needle biopsy*.

fluoride   A mineral primarily used for dental health that can interfere with your thyroid's production of hormones. Fluoride can cause or worsen hypothyroidism, but is an inexpensive and relatively harmless remedy for hyperthyroidism (either by itself, or combined with medication such as Tapazole).

follicular thyroid cancer   The second most common form of thyroid cancer, accounting for about 12 percent of cases. Its cure rate is 97 percent. See also *thyroid cancer*.

free T3   The amount of T3 in your bloodstream that's available for powering up your cells (as opposed to the T3 that's rendered inert by being bound by proteins). Measuring free T3 is one of the key ways to determine your thyroid's status.

free T4   The amount of T4 in your bloodstream that's available for conversion to T3 (as opposed to the T4 that's rendered inert by being bound by proteins). Measuring free T4 is one of the key ways to determine your thyroid's status.

ghrelin   A hormone produced by cells in your stomach and pancreas that makes you hungry. When you skimp on sleep your body produces more ghrelin, making it likelier that you'll overeat. See also *leptin*.

glandular thyroid   See *desiccated thyroid*.

glucose   A fundamental sugar your body creates from the food you eat. The mitochondria in your cells convert it into energy.

goiter   A large non-cancerous growth on your thyroid, typically resulting from a lack of iodine or hyperthyroidism.

goitrogens   Foods that inhibit your thyroid's ability to make its hormones and so can combat hyperthyroidism. These include cruciferous vegetables such as broccoli, cauliflower, cabbage, Brussels sprouts, and kale, which are all loaded with indole-3-carbinol; and soy products, which contain isoflavones.

Graves' disease   An autoimmune disease in which your immune system mistakes your thyroid for a threat and attacks it with TSI antibodies. Over 80 percent of hyperthyroidism cases are caused by Graves' disease.

Hashimoto's disease   An autoimmune disease in which your immune system mistakes your thyroid for a threat and attacks it with antibodies. Roughly 75-85 percent of hypothyroidism cases are caused by Hashimoto's disease.

Hashitoxicosis   A manifestation of Hashimoto's disease that swings you back and forth between hyperthyroidism (during antibody attacks that slaughter thyroid cells, spilling out their stored hormones) and hypothyroidism (between attacks, as the thyroid becomes increasingly less functional). These extreme states can average out, making your TSH appear normal.

high-intensity interval training   See *burst training*.

hot nodule   See *thyroid nodule*.

hyperthyroid eye disease   Ocular problems from hyperthyroidism, and especially Graves' disease, including "lid lag," sensitivity to light, feeling painful dryness or grittiness in the eyes, double vision, and eyelids retracting while the eyes enlarge and protrude to create a "bug-eyed" look.

hyperthyroidism   A disease that causes your thyroid to produce too much of its hormones, leading to dangerous overstimulation of your body's cells. Common symptoms include a pounding heart, anxiety, panic attacks, tremors, and goiters.

hypothalamus   The portion of your brain that (among other things) senses when your body needs more energy and sends a chemical signal to your pituitary gland to make more TSH.

hypothyroidism   A disease in which you don't have enough thyroid hormones to provide your body's cells with the energy they need. Common symptoms include fatigue, weight gain, depression, slowed thinking, and hair loss. Experts estimate 1 in 10 Americans suffers from hypothyroidism.

indole-3-carbinol   A natural compound found in cruciferous vegetables—such as broccoli, cauliflower, cabbage, Brussels sprouts, and kale—that can interfere with your thyroid's hormone production and so may be useful in combating hyperthyroidism.

insulin resistance   A condition in which your cell receptors designed to respond to insulin become less sensitive, requiring your body to pump out significantly more insulin than normal. This can lead to decreased fat burning, increased inflammation, and diseases such as high blood pressure. You can potentially re-sensitive the cell receptors by taking *conjugated linoleic acid (CLA)* and/or *lipoic acid.*

inulin   A natural fiber extracted from plants such as Jerusalem artichoke, wild yam, and chicory. Once hard to find, inulin is now readily available in powder form via the commercial product Metamucil Clear & Natural. Inulin dissolves completely in water, and is very mildly sweet, so you can add it to smoothies, oatmeal, etc., and barely notice it's there. See also *PGX.*

iodine   The element your thyroid combines with tyrosine to make its hormones.

iodine uptake and thyroid scan   Test that involves injecting you with or having you swallow a tiny amount of radioactive iodine, waiting 6-24 hours, and then scanning your neck to get a clear picture of what's happening in your thyroid.

iodine-induced thyroiditis   See *thyroiditis.*

isoflavones   A natural compound found in soy products that can interfere with your thyroid's hormone production and so may be useful in combating hyperthyroidism.

isthmus   The middle section of your thyroid, connecting its left and right lobes.

IU/mL   International unit for antibodies per milliliter of blood, used to measure TPO and Tg antibodies.

kava-kava   A natural remedy that may help calm anxiety due to hyperthyroidism. See also *theanine* and *benzodiazepines.*

L-carnitine   An amino acid that can help fight hyperthyroidism by interfering with T3's ability to penetrate cell membranes and the thyroid's responsiveness to TSH. L-carnitine is inexpensive, readily available, and has virtually no side effects.

lean body mass (LBM)   The parts of your body that are fat-free, including your muscles and bones.

leptin   A hormone that decreases appetite. When you skimp on sleep your body produces less leptin, making it likelier that you'll overeat. See also *ghrelin.*

Levothroid   Thyroid medication that's a synthetic version of T4, manufactured by Forest Laboratories (FRX.com). The generic version is levothyroxine.

levothyroxine   Thyroid medication that's a synthetic version of T4. The most prescribed brand name version is Synthroid.

Levoxyl   Thyroid medication that's a synthetic version of T4, manufactured by King Pharmaceuticals (KingPharm.com). The generic version is levothyroxine.

liothyronine   Thyroid medication that's a synthetic version of T3. The brand name version is Cytomel.

lipoic acid   A natural dietary supplement that can help combat *insulin resistance* by re-sensitizing insulin cell receptors. See also *conjugated linoleic acid (CLA)*.

lobes   The left and right parts of your thyroid gland. If one lobe fails or is removed, the other can take over the job of making hormones.

low stomach acid   A condition that can be caused by age, stress, and/or food sensitivity. It decreases your stomach's ability to digest protein, making less protein available to build muscle. It also creates the possibility of bacterial overgrowth in the small intestine, which can lead to your body extracting more calories from the foods you eat and storing them as fat. A telltale sign of the latter is continual bloating. Your doctor can check for such overgrowth via a urine organic acid test for gut *dysbiosis* (meaning "out of balance"). See also *betaine HCl*.

magnesium   A natural remedy for a rapid heartbeat due to hyperthyroidism.

mcg   Short for microgram.

medullary thyroid cancer   The third most common form of thyroid cancer, accounting for about 5 percent of cases. The recommended treatment is surgically removing the entire thyroid, possibly the lymph nodes, and anywhere else it appears to have invaded.

MEN1 syndrome   Multiple endocrine neoplasia 1, a rare condition in which several different endocrine glands—the thyroid, parathyroids, pancreas, pituitary, and/or adrenals—start growing tumors at the same time. These tumors usually aren't cancerous, but they lead to an overproduction of hormones. Also known as Werner's syndrome.

MEN2 syndrome   Multiple endocrine neoplasia 2, a rare condition in which several different endocrine glands start growing cancerous tumors at the same time. Also known as Sipple syndrome.

metabolism   Your body's energy level, which is set by your hypothalamus and enforced by your thyroid's hormones.

methimazole   Medication that very effectively combats even severe hyperthyroidism by interfering with the thyroid's ability to make its hormones. The brand name version is Tapazole.

mg   Short for milligram. Equivalent to 1,000 mcg.

mitochondria   The "power plants" in each of your cells that take glucose and convert it into energy, or ATP.

mIU/L   Milli-international units per liter of blood, used to measure TSH.

mono-iodothyronine   See *T1*.

multiple endocrine neoplasia 1   See *MEN1 syndrome*.

multiple endocrine neoplasia 2   See *MEN2 syndrome*.

natural desiccated thyroid   See *desiccated thyroid*.

Nature-Throid   Medication made from desiccated pig thyroid that contains all four thyroid hormones: T4, T3, T2, and T1. Manufactured by RLC Labs (RLCLabs. com). This medication is identical to RLC's WesThroid.

NDT   See *desiccated thyroid*.

ng/dL   Nanograms per deciliter of blood, used to measure free T4.

nodule   See *thyroid nodule*.

nori   A seaweed that's an excellent source of iodine.

painful subacute thyroiditis   See *thyroiditis*.

papillary thyroid cancer   The most common form of thyroid cancer, accounting for about 80 percent of cases. It's typically caused by exposure to radiation. Its cure rate is 97 percent. See also *thyroid cancer*.

parathyroid glands   Small glands residing behind your thyroid that regulate the amount of calcium in your blood and bones.

pg/dL   Picograms per deciliter of blood, used to measure free T3.

PGX   PolyGlycopleX, a natural fiber extracted from plants. PGX absorbs a great deal of water and so is especially good at filling you up if you take it right before a meal. PGX is readily available commercially in both capsule and softgel forms. See also *inulin*.

pheochromocytoma   A condition in which your adrenal glands' cells spawn tumors that grow either on the glands or outside of them, and produce hormones independently, resulting in too much cortisol. See also *Cushing's syndrome*.

pituitary disease   Underactivity or overactivity of the pituitary glands, most commonly caused by one or more tumors. If a pituitary tumor is 14 millimeters or smaller, it can usually be shrunk with the medicine bromocriptine. Otherwise, surgery is required.

pituitary gland   A pea-size organ just above your sinuses that, among other things, regulates the hormone production of your thyroid (via TSH) and adrenal glands (via ACTH).

Plummer's disease   The second most common cause of hyperthyroidism, resulting in one or more non-cancerous nodules that produce hormones independently— without waiting to be stimulated by TSH. Also called Plummer's adenoma (when there's just one nodule) or toxic multinodular goiter.

PolyGlycopleX   See *PGX*.

postpartum thyroiditis   See *thyroiditis*.

propranolol   A beta blocker that's effective at slowing a rapid heartbeat caused by hyperthyroidism.

PTU (propylthiouracil)   Medication that combats hyperthyroidism by interfering with the thyroid's ability to make its hormones. PTU has largely been replaced by the superior medication Tapazole, but is useful if you're allergic to Tapazole, find Tapazole ineffective, or are pregnant.

radioiodine ablation   A procedure designed to end hyperthyroidism via radioactive iodine that destroys a substantial percentage of the thyroid's cells, making it too small to continue overproducing hormones. This procedure is also used to destroy remaining thyroid cells after the thyroid is removed (typically due to cancer).

red blood cell element test   Measures your three-month average levels of essential chemicals boron, chromium, calcium, copper, iron, magnesium, manganese, molybdenum, phosphorus, potassium, selenium, vanadium, and zinc; and detects the presence of the toxins arsenic, cadmium, lead, mercury, and thallium.

resting metabolic rate (RMR)   A measure of your base level of activity (your heart beating, your lungs breathing, your brain processing information, etc.) when you're not doing anything strenuous.

reverse T3   A nonfunctional thyroid hormone your body creates by removing an iodine atom from obsolete or excess T4. The resulting reverse T3 can then be easily flushed from your system.

RMR   See *resting metabolic rate.*

salivary cortisol testing   A test in which you take a sample of your saliva periodically over 24 hours, which allows your doctor to track your cortisol levels throughout the day. See also *cortisol challenge test.*

selenium   The chemical your body uses to make the enzyme deiodinase type 1 effective. You can ensure you have enough selenium by eating a single Brazil nut a day.

shoulder stand   Yoga posture in which you lie flat on your back, letting your body rest on your shoulders and the back of your neck, and raise your legs together until they're pointing straight up. This places substantial compression on your thyroid and can increase the blood supply to it.

silent thyroiditis   See *thyroiditis.*

Sipple syndrome   See *MEN2 syndrome.*

Stevia   A natural sugar substitute you can use in place of unhealthy artificial sweeteners. See also *Xylitol.*

strength training   A workout method that builds up your muscles, which in turn helps you burn fat by both raising your metabolism and heightening your body's responsiveness to insulin. Strength training works best when combined with *burst training.*

struma ovarii   A rare condition in which thyroid cells grow in the ovaries. If these cells produce hormones independently, they'll make you hyperthyroid. They're treated via surgical removal.

Synthroid   Bestselling thyroid medication that's a synthetic version of T4, manufactured by Abbott (Abbott.com). The generic version is levothyroxine.

T1   A thyroid hormone with one iodine atom. No useful function has been discovered for T1 so far, but that may change with further research. Also called mono-iodothyronine.

T2   A thyroid hormone with two iodine atoms that studies have found plays a role in metabolism and burning fat. Also called do-iodothyronine.

T3   A thyroid hormone with three iodine atoms that does the work of powering up the mitochondria in your cells. Also called tri-iodothyronine. Taking T3 medication can be especially effective in lifting depression.

T4   A thyroid hormone with four iodine atoms designed to circulate in your bloodstream, and be stored in your tissues, until it's needed to be converted into T3. Also called thyroxine or tetra-iodothyronine.

Tanita Segmental scale   A high-tech scale that identifies how much fat you have and where it's located on your body.

Tapazole   Medication that very effectively combats even severe hyperthyroidism by interfering with the thyroid's ability to make its hormones. The generic version is methimazole.

tetra-iodothyronine   See *T4*.

Tg   Thyroglobulin antibodies, which attack your thyroid and cause the autoimmune disease Hashimoto's.

theanine   A natural remedy which may help calm anxiety due to hyperthyroidism. See also *kava-kava* and *benzodiazepines*.

thyroglobulin   The protein your thyroid binds with iodine to make its hormones.

thyroglobulin antibodies   See *Tg*.

thyroid   A butterfly-shaped gland that resides in your neck. It produces T4, T3, T2, and T1 hormones that regulate the energy level, growth, and reproduction of every cell in your body.

thyroid cancer   A serious but seldom fatal disease that's typically treated with surgery and radioactive iodine. The most common forms are papillary and follicular, which have a cure rate of 97 percent.

thyroid disease   A medical condition of your thyroid, such as hypothyroidism, hyperthyroidism, or thyroid cancer.

thyroid eye disease   See *hyperthyroid eye disease*.

thyroid nodule   A small growth on your thyroid. If a scan indicates the nodule is "cold," meaning it's not absorbing iodine and or making hormones, there's about a 10 percent chance it's cancerous. Alternatively, if the nodule is "hot," it's producing hormones and may be making you hyperthyroid.

thyroid peroxidase antibodies   See *TPO*.

thyroid scan   See *iodine uptake* and *thyroid scan*.

thyroid stimulating hormone   See *TSH*.

thyroid stimulating immunoglobulin   See *TSI*.

thyroid storm   A condition in which you're so overloaded with thyroid hormones that you're at risk of a heart attack. The quickest way to end this condition is to overload you with iodine, which "blows a fuse" and temporarily shuts down your thyroid.

thyroiditis   A condition in which antibodies attack and inflame your thyroid. This usually stems from Hashitoxicosis, but can also result from (typically) temporary illnesses such as painful subacute thyroiditis (triggered by a respiratory infection), silent thyroiditis (which causes no pain), postpartum thyroiditis (which occurs after pregnancy), and iodine-induced thyroiditis (which is caused by iodine overdosing).

Thyrolar   Thyroid medication that's a synthetic mix of T4 and T3 in a 4:1 ratio. Manufactured by Forest Laboratories (FRX.com).

thyrotoxicosis factitia   A condition in which hyperthyroidism occurs as a result of artificial rather than natural causes—such as an overdose of thyroid medication.

thyroxine   See *T4*.

TOFI   Thin outside, fat inside. To avoid becoming TOFI, focus on shedding fat rather than just weight.

total T3   The total amount of T3 in your body—that is, both free T3 and the T3 bound by proteins. This information seldom has practical value, as what matters is free T3.

total T4   The total amount of T4 in your body—that is, both free T4 and the T4 bound by proteins. This information seldom has practical value, as what matters is free T4.

toxic nodule   A small non-cancerous growth that produces thyroid hormones independently. This is a result of Plummer's disease.

TPO   Thyroid peroxidase antibodies, which attack your thyroid and cause the autoimmune disease Hashimoto's.

tri-iodothyronine   See *T3*.

TSH   Thyroid stimulating hormone, made by your pituitary gland to instruct your thyroid gland to increase its T4, T3, T2, and T2 production. Measuring your TSH level (which is a 2-3 month average) is one of the key ways to determine your thyroid's status.

TSH-secreting pituitary adenoma   See *pituitary disease.*

TSI   Thyroid stimulating immunoglobulin, which are antibodies that attack your thyroid and cause the autoimmune disease Graves'.

tyrosine   The amino acid your thyroid combines with iodine to make its hormones.

ultrasound   Safe and inexpensive test that can create images of your thyroid by bouncing high-frequency sound waves off it.

Unithroid   Thyroid medication that's a synthetic version of T4, manufactured by Jerome Stevens Pharmaceuticals (Unithroid.com). The generic version is levothyroxine.

wakame   A seaweed that's an excellent source of iodine.

Werner's syndrome   See *MEN1 syndrome.*

WesThroid   Medication made from desiccated pig thyroid that contains all four thyroid hormones: T4, T3, T2, and T1. Manufactured by RLC Labs (RLCLabs. com). This medication is identical to RLC's Nature-Throid.

Xylitol   A natural sugar substitute you can use in place of unhealthy artificial sweeteners. See also *Stevia.*

Resources

There are a number of organizations and websites available to help you locate the right doctor, learn more about thyroid disease, research thyroid medications, and live a healthier life. This appendix describes some of the very best of these information sources.

Also be sure to visit this book's own website at CIGThyroid.com, which provides clickable links to all the resources in this appendix—and more—sparing you from having to type in lots of web addresses.

Finding the Right Doctor

Finding a doctor who's highly skilled and yet willing to collaborate with you on your diagnosis and treatment isn't always easy. The following organizations and websites will help. Except for MyFax.com, these sites are all free.

In addition, take care to read Chapters 3 and 4, which explain what to seek and what to avoid in a thyroid doctor.

American Medical Association's DoctorFinder
Web: AMA-assn.org/aps/amahg.htm
This comprehensive site lists virtually every licensed doctor in the United States—over 814,000 physicians. You can search by location, name, and/or specialty (choose the *Endocrinology, Diabetes, and Metabolism* option).

American Association of Clinical Endocrinologists
Web: AACE.com/resources/memsearch.php
This professional organization for endocrinologists will let you search for its U.S. and international members based on location and specialty (choose the *Thyroid Dysfunction* option).

American Association of Naturopathic Physicians

Web: Naturopathic.org

This professional organization consists of alternative health practitioners who "teach their patients to use diet, exercise, lifestyle changes, and cutting-edge natural therapies to enhance their bodies' ability to ward off and combat disease," and who "blend the best of modern medical science and traditional natural medical approaches to not only treat disease but also restore health." If you want to be assured that your request for desiccated thyroid won't lead to a confrontation with your physician, click this site's *Find a Doctor* link to search by name, location, or specialty (choose either the *Adrenal Fatigue/Endocrinology* or *Chronic Fatigue/Autoimmune Disorders* option).

Thyroid Top Doctors

Web: Thyroid-info.com/topdrs

Author and patient advocate Mary Shomon runs this site listing U.S. thyroid doctors nominated by her readers. According to Shomon, a top physician is "a doctor who listens, cares, has an open mind, wants us to understand and participate in our treatment decisions, and isn't beholden to a particular drug company." Included are endocrinologists, thyroid specialists, thyroid surgeons, integrative physicians, and more. First click on your state, and then scroll through the list to find doctors in your city.

American Board of Medical Specialties

Web: ABMS.org

If you want to check on whether a U.S. doctor you're considering is board certified in his or her specialty, click the *Is Your Doctor Certified?* link, follow the instructions for free registration, and then provide your doctor's name.

Integrative Health Care

Web: IntegrativeHealthCare.com

If you live in or near Scottsdale, Arizona, you may want to consider seeing Dr. Alan Christianson, who's the co-author of this book. Integrative Health Care is Alan's clinic. You can learn about Alan's background and read patient testimonials at CIGThyroid.com/alan.htm.

MyFax
Web: MyFax.com
One of the ways to get involved with your thyroid care is to have your doctor's office fax you the results of your thyroid blood tests. If you don't have a fax machine, you can get faxes e-mailed to you as PDF attachments. An especially good and inexpensive service for the latter is MyFax.com, which is free for a 30-day trial period, and then $10 a month (covering up to 200 pages received and 100 sent per month). For additional details, visit MyFax.com/pricing.aspx.

Learning More About Thyroid Disease

We've tried to cover everything you're likely to need to know about thyroid disease in this book, but there may be times when you require additional information. You can use the following websites—including the official site for this book—to fill in further details and/or breaking news. Except for UpToDate.com, these sites are all free.

***The Complete Idiot's Guide to Thyroid Disease* Website**
Web: CIGThyroid.com
CIGThyroid.com is the official website for this book. It lists all the resources in this appendix (and more) as clickable links, sparing you from having to type a lot of web addresses. It also features updates, discounts, and other extras. Please feel encouraged to visit it monthly.

Thyroid Disease Manager
Web: ThyroidManager.org
This excellent site is written by doctors and for doctors. It's quite technical, so if jargon makes you uncomfortable, steer clear. Otherwise, you can find a wealth of information here focused directly on thyroid disease.

UpToDate
Web: UpToDate.com
This high-quality collection of medical articles is written and peer reviewed by doctors, and is also targeted primarily at doctors. However, the writing is better and easier to understand than that of most medical journals; plus, as its name implies, it's frequently updated. If you can deal with the scientific details, the site is a great resource for in-depth information on virtually any medical topic—which is why it has an audience of nearly 400,000. Patient-level information (at UpToDate.com/patients) is free. If you need more detailed technical information, you can buy full access to the site for a week—long enough to research any pressing medical question—for under $20.

Thyroid-Info.com and **About.com: Thyroid Disease**
Web: Thyroid-Info.com and Thyroid.about.com
Author and thyroid health advocate Mary Shomon runs both of these sites, offering helpful information written from a patient's perspective.

PubMed
Web: PubMed.gov
The U.S. Government's National Institutes of Health run this invaluable site, which is a clearinghouse for virtually all published medical research—including studies of thyroid disease. The material is as technical as it gets, but if you need to perform cutting-edge research, this is the place to start. To learn more, click the home page's *Help* link.

Medline Plus
Web: MedlinePlus.gov
The U.S. Government's National Institutes of Health also run this site, which—in contrast to PubMed—is designed to be patient friendly. It provides a great deal of solid information about all major illnesses, including thyroid disease.

American Cancer Society and **OncoLink**
Web: Cancer.org and OncoLink.org
As a supplement to Chapter 13, you may want to visit the websites of two superb cancer organizations. The American Cancer Society has a booklet about thyroid cancer at www.cancer.org/Cancer/ThyroidCancer/index, and OncoLink has an excellent detailed article on the subject at OncoLink.org/types/section.cfm?c=7&s=26.

Thyroid Cancer Survivors' Association
Web: ThyCa.org
Information about both thyroid cancer and support groups for those struck by the disease can be found at this site run by thyroid cancer survivors since 1995.

Thyroid Medication Manufacturers

If you're trying to decide which thyroid medications to choose (as discussed in Chapters 3 and 8), you may find it useful to explore the websites of their manufacturers. They are as follows:

Synthroid (Abbott)
Web: Abbott.com

Cytomel and Levoxyl (King Pharmaceuticals)
Web: KingPharm.com

Unithroid (Jerome Stevens Pharmaceuticals)
Web: Unithroid.com

Nature-Throid and WesThroid (RLC Labs)
Web: RLCLabs.com

Armour Thyroid, Thyrolar, and Levothroid (Forest Laboratories)
Web: ArmourThyroid.com and FRX.com

Desiccated Thyroid Powder (American Laboratories)
(This is the raw material for Nature-Throid, WesThroid, Armour Thyroid, etc.)
Web: AmericanLaboratories.com

Lifestyle & Diet Help

As explained in Chapters 18-21, both your thyroid's health and your overall health
will be improved if you avoid toxins and eat right. The following are some of the
finest resources to help you go green and organic … and to lose weight while you're
at it.

Environmental Working Group
Web: EWG.org
Founded in 1993, EWG is a nonprofit group devoted to protecting consumers from
environmental toxins—the cause of most thyroid disease. Its site provides numerous tips on how to avoid food pesticides, poisons in cosmetics, and other chemical
dangers.

Green Guide for Everyday Living
Web: TheGreenGuide.com
This site from the National Geographic Society is filled with simple tips that "make
going green a gradual and affordable process rather than an all-or-nothing plunge."
Click the *Go Local* option to find organic and "green" companies in your area.

Local Harvest and USDA Agricultural Marketing Service
Web: LocalHarvest.org and Apps.ams.usda.gov/FarmersMarkets
Use these wonderful sites to find local family farms and farmers' markets, which are
often the best sources for inexpensive organic food.

Eatwild

Web: Eatwild.com

Use this site to locate pasture-based farms near you that sell grass-fed meat and dairy products.

MyFoodDiary

Web: MyFoodDiary.com

The chances are you'll eat less and lose weight if you keep track of what you consume. This website makes it easy to do so, employing a database of over 70,000 foods. It also provides an exercise log that calculates the calories burned for over 700 activities, creates reports that gently encourage you to keep losing (and discourage you from gaining), and hosts hundreds of forums for online group support. It costs $9 a month.

CalorieKing

Web: CalorieKing.com

Like MyFoodDiary, this site helps you track your eating via an extensive food database and provides support via online communities. It also offers tutorials and tips that help guide you to lose weight. It costs $12 a month.

Weight Watchers

Web: WeightWatchers.com

The renowned Weight Watchers program was designed for live meetings, and that's still how it works best. This site lets you discover when and where meetings are taking place near you.

J. J. Virgin

Web: JJVirgin.com

Fitness and nutrition guru J. J. Virgin has helped such celebrities as Ben Stiller, Janeane Garofalo, Gene Simmons, Brandon Routh, and mega-selling author Jack Canfield, and for two years was the nutrition expert on the *Dr. Phil* show. Chapter 20 of this book is devoted to Virgin's advice on shedding fat. In addition to personal coaching, Virgin offers various products through her website—including her book *Six Weeks to Sleeveless and Sexy*.

Index

Numbers

Q-R

X-Y-Z